NURSING PARTNERSHIP

A Model for Nursing Practice

Judith Christensen RCpN BA MSc(App) PhD
Head, School of Nursing, Health and Environmental Sciences,
Wellington Polytechnic,
Wellington, New Zealand

Foreword by
Margaret F. Alexander BSc PhD RGN SCM RNT FRCN
Professor and Head, Department of Health and Nursing Studies,
Glasgow Caledonian University,
Glasgow, UK

CHURCHILL LIVINGSTONE
EDINBURGH LONDON MADRID MELBOURNE NEW YORK AND TOKYO 1993

CHURCHILL LIVINGSTONE
Medical Division of Longman Group UK Limited

Distributed in the United States of America by
Churchill Livingstone Inc., 650 Avenue of the Americas,
New York, N.Y. 10011, and by associated companies,
branches and representatives throughout the world.

First edition 1990: Daphne Brasell Associates Press
UK edition 1993: Longman Group UK Limited

ISBN 0-443-04934-3

British Library of Cataloguing in Publication Data
A catalogue record for this book is available from the British Library.

Library of Congress Cataloging in Publication Data
A catalog record for this book is available from the Library of Congress.

Designed by Margaret Cochran
Typeset by Wordset Enterprises Ltd, Wellington
Film-making by the Government Printer, Wellington,
New Zealand

The
publisher's
policy is to use
paper manufactured
from sustainable forests

Produced by Longman Singapore (Pte) Ltd
Printed in Singapore

CONTENTS

FOREWORD

This is a book for our time – a deeply searching, challenging, courageous book which systematically examines, analyses and illuminates in detail the day to day reality of nursing. But here there is no narrow focus, no introspective musing. The turbulent, restless and highly complex context of the society, the culture and the health care delivery system within which nursing, the interaction between nurses and patients or clients, is practised, is kept ever before the reader. Were it not for the fact that the author very clearly refers to New Zealand as the context for her research, the reader could be forgiven for thinking it had originated in the United Kingdom. The issues, at macro and micro level, are identical. Thus, the conceptual model for nursing care which Judith Christensen discovers – and which she continues to refine and develop – has great potential, not only to advance our knowledge of the specific contribution of nursing to the outcomes of care but to encourage productive reflection on nursing practice. Its potential is wider than nursing. Other members of the health care team would also find the model applicable in their practice.

For those nurses who feel somewhat sceptical of nursing theories and models, and who see them as remote from practice, this book should be a turning point, because the Nursing Partnership model will ring true. It is derived directly from practice. For all nurses, educators and researchers, the book is a rich source of information – about the partnership between the provider and the consumer of nursing care, about the application of grounded theory in nursing research, about consistency in the interpretation of a philosophy.

Judith Christensen's keen and expert nursing observation of two patients, whose vivid vignettes capture the reader's attention from the commencement of the book, is the trigger for her research question – 'What is happening here?' What follows as that question is explored in all its many facets is the illumination of a passage, a shared journey, as nurse and patient, from their different perspectives, work their way together through a health-related experience. The work of the patient/client and the work of the nurse are articulated in their own words, as they negotiate their separate preparations for entry to this passage and their partnership throughout, until the leaving point is reached. Judith Christensen's analytic skills, her creative induction using grounded theory and the depth of her nursing experience have enabled her to elucidate key concepts which, uniquely I believe at this point, highlight the fact that this is not only a partnership, but a working partnership, the complex dimensions of which are set within the important contextual determinants which the client, the nurse, and the community's culture, beliefs, values and health care system contribute.

In her journey towards her conceptualisation of the giving and receiving of nursing care as a partnership, Judith Christensen is not afraid to expose deficiencies in care as well as strengths. For example, she found nurses had only a limited awareness of the importance to patients of their 'comforting' role, particularly when it was beneficial, and that they tended to undervalue this aspect of care. They also failed to use problems they had identified as a basis for planning nursing care. There were also however examples of excellence. These points are richly illustrated in the data.

There is a realistic dynamism about this book and all it explains. There is no prescribed end point; no sense that this is the complete answer. The model was developed in the context of acute care in a surgical ward. It was revised, to take into account the views of colleagues, and the different partnerships, the different health-related experiences and contexts which pertain in community care settings. The use of the model in nursing practice and in nurse education is described, but, in harmony with the philosophy of partnership, the author never prescribes. She simply illustrates the implications of using the nursing partnership model. For example, in curriculum development and delivery, the passage of the student would reflect both giving and receiving; a partnership, composed of her own work, the work of the educator and the work of the role model practising nurse.

The values and ethic of a true scholar are reflected in Judith Christensen's invitation to nurses to join her on her voyage of discovery; to feel that the model which she has created belongs to them, and to share in its further development. She encourages nurses to use it, reflecting particularly on the contextual determinants which may be significant locally, to experiment with it and to modify it so that it works for them and for their patients, clients or students.

Nothing is finite in the Nursing Partnership. There is no prescription – no ready made documentation – but a clear message that *nursing matters*. I personally feel that, if we believe in a true partnership in care, we have a responsibility to examine this model intently. It speaks to me of values which I think are fundamental to nursing. I hope it will be used, shared and further developed, in response to Judith Christensen's invitation.

1993

M.F.A

PREFACE

1990 is a very special year. Throughout the world barriers which have served to control people, at individual and state level, are being broken down; oppression is being challenged on a wide front; justice is being claimed; people are asserting their right to choose; more collegial relationships are being sought to replace those which have been characterised by the domination of one person or people by another.

In Aotearoa-New Zealand we are commemorating the signing of the Treaty of Waitangi which took place in 1840. This year, in the context of a changing world, the majority European community and institutions are being challenged to acknowledge anew the fundamental equity inherent within the treaty relationship with the tangata whenua, the Maori people. At last, diversity is beginning to be valued rather than feared; power is starting to be shared; there is an increasing acknowledgement of the legitimate claims of the Maori people – the tangata whenua; and there is an emergent hope that equality, justice and autonomy will prevail.

Many New Zealanders of European heritage are finding it very difficult to accept that the Maori people have suffered in any way from the imposition of a foreign culture. Reactions of anger and/or confusion, and even fear, are common when faced with many accusations such as those so clearly implied in the following two examples.

> Kei muri i te awe kapara he tangata ke, mana te ao, he ma.
> Shadowed behind the tatooed face a stranger stands, he owns the earth, and he is white. (an ancestral saying)

> But I am constantly reminded of the number of Pakeha people who know better than I do what is good for me. It is about time we were allowed to think for ourselves and to say which things we want and why we want them. And to say that we do things for our reasons and not for the reasons set down by Pakeha experts. (Rangihau, 1975, p 232)

It is a time for reaching out and listening to the views of others, and revising many relationships. This is occurring on a wider front than between the people of different cultures. Within the health-care field the traditional doctor-nurse relationship is being similarly challenged. In a recent article three American doctors suggest that nursing's quest for autonomy 'is an extension of the civil rights movement and more particularly the women's movement' (Stein, Watts and Howell, 1990, p 547). They go on to make a statement that has wider relevance.

> Physicians for the most part did not perceive nurses to be subservient in the first place and are thus confused by their efforts to gain equality. It is, of course, not unusual for those in power to be oblivious to the fact that those under them may feel oppressed. (ibid, p 548)

Nurses are seeking a collegial partnership in health care with their medical and other peers. The word 'partnership' is an appropriate word to use when it is defined as an alliance between two or more people involved in a shared venture. There is no doubt that people enter into many different kinds of partnerships during their lifetime. These vary from formal ones, such as treaties, business or marriage contracts, to informal ones, such as friendships. The use of a partnership framework redefines any relationship to one where it is assumed that both participants are active, both recognise their rights and obligations, and each has a role to play to achieve a negotiated outcome.

The relationship between a consumer and the provider of a service is now increasingly portrayed as a partnership. Previously such services were often supplied within a paternalistic framework where the expert, seemingly with the best of intentions, made decisions for consumers while usually denying them information, individual responsibility and the right to choose.

Perhaps the archetypal relationship of this kind has been that of doctor and patient. Nursing, too, is not immune to accusations of involvement in this pattern of autocratic behaviour. One commonly portrayed image of nursing is that of a 'bossy' nurse using military-like protocols to demand total obedience from junior staff and patients alike. However, consumers of health and other services are beginning to challenge this pattern of perceived subserviance and are being encouraged to assert their rights — particularly the right to know and the right to choose.

In her report on the cervical cancer inquiry Judge Cartwright reflected this change.

> Although decisions about treatment can never be transferred totally to the patient, the responsibility is shared if the doctor knows that the patient understands the nature of her condition and the treatment available and is a willing participant. (Cartwright, 1988, p 158)

Against this local and international background of changing relationships at many levels, the theoretical framework of the Nursing Partnership has been generated from research data using the grounded theory method. As the field data (mostly interviews with patients and nurses in a number of surgical wards) were analysed, the mutual activity of patient and nurse became apparent. There was no denying that both had their own work to do to assist the patient/person to get through a particular experience. This was indeed a partnership of experts.

Stevens gave encouragement by her use of the term.

> For me, the partnership between patient and nurse must be reflected in a theory that allows each to bring his particular expertise, while fully utilising the expertness of the other. (Stevens, 1979, p 261)

Much blood, sweat and tears were shed before the Nursing Partnership model took shape and the doctoral dissertation which gave rise to this book was completed. Nursing colleagues expressed the view that the product of the research was thought-provoking and perhaps timely in view of the current upheaval in the nursing practice environment. It is a positive assertion of the valuable contribution nursing can make to improve the lives of people. Even while it is still changing and developing, the framework challenges nurses to think anew about their practice; the nurse administrator to rethink the organisation of nursing care; the teacher to visualise new ways of presenting nursing to those entering the profession; and the researcher to devise studies which confirm and expand the emergent theory.

In the account of the Nursing Partnership which follows there is an orderly sequence. The *Introduction* sets the scene by briefly describing the background to the original research. *Chapter 1* places the theoretical framework in a broader nursing context with selective use of nursing and related literature. In *Chapter 2* the theory is introduced. *Chapter 3* presents the Beginning – the first stage of the person's passage of receiving nursing through a health-related experience within the Nursing Partnership. In *Chapter 4*, the second stage – Entering the Nursing Partnership: Settling In – is discussed with the focus on the work of both patient and nurse. *Chapters 5 and 6* contain detailed discussion on the critical third stage – Negotiating the Nursing Partnership. The work of the patient is presented in the first of these chapters, and the work of the nurse in the second. *Chapter 7* presents a discussion on the last stage – Leaving the Nursing Partnership: Going Home – and includes a description of the work of both patient and nurse. *Chapter 8* completes the presentation of the theoretical framework with the focus moving to the determinants which directly affect the shape of the passage and the partnership.

Since completion of the study that generated the grounded theory of the Nursing Partnership, the model has undergone a process of review and further development and this modified version is presented in *Chapter 9*.

Chapters 10 and 11 discuss the possible application of the Nursing Partnership model for nursing practice and education.

The book concludes with a short summary and a discussion on the future of the evolving theory in *Chapter 12*. The appendices present the research study which generated the grounded theory.

As with any study of this nature, the work is incomplete. Such a voyage of discovery often raises more questions than it answers. As the writing progressed, further development of the framework took place, and this evolutionary process will continue.

The inevitable unfinished nature of this kind of theorising is acknowledged by Meleis when she comments:

> At some point, a project needs to be abandoned so that others in the field will have a chance to play with its ideas in order to modify, extend, refine, or refute their own . . . . The reader is urged to consider that this project is intentionally an incomplete-completed project, a temporarily abandoned project that represents the thinking and the analysis of one author, seen through her own 'wide-lensed glasses' at a certain point in time. (Meleis, 1985, p 4)

If this book makes nurses feel good about themselves and their role, if it helps nurses to hold their heads high and courageously assert their invaluable contribution to the health of the community; if people benefit by receiving quality nursing during a health experience, then the personal investment in the research, the thesis writing and the rewriting for publication has been well worthwhile.

ACKNOWLEDGEMENTS

The study on which this book is based would not have been possible without the willing participation of the special people who were undergoing surgery at the time of the research. Without exception they welcomed me and generously shared their experience.

Nursing administration personnel gave me support and encouragement throughout the study and the nursing staff in the five wards used in the study willingly gave their assistance throughout the time in the field.

During the course of the study both of my parents were very ill. Their hospital and illness experiences, while personally distressing, helped me to gain new and valuable insights into the meaning of the field data. I am saddened that my mother did not live to read the outcome.

Without the discernment and persistence of Norma Chick, the experienced wisdom of Ray Adams, and the early encouragement of Nan Kinross, all educators at Massey University, I would have found it difficult to complete the research and thesis.

Two years of full-time study was made possible by awards from the Department of Education, the British War Memorial Nurses' Fund and the Nursing Education and Research Foundation. NERF has continued its support in the brave decision to sponsor the publication of this book. Throughout its history NERF has been a constant proponent of the continuing development of the profession during a period of dramatic change in, and constant challenge to, nursing in New Zealand.

Completing this work has necessitated my spending many many hours alone. During these times Kermit and Jessica were quietly and lovingly there. Anxiety was kept more or less under control by my daily walks with Kermit over the hills and on the beaches around Island Bay.

The further development of the model from the thesis to its form in this book has been a project shared with my colleagues and the students of the Wellington Polytechnic School of Nursing and

Health Education as we have worked on the development of a curriculum based on the Nursing Partnership. I am particularly indebted to Annette Stevenson, Fran Richardson and Rose McEldowney for their assistance with the further development of the Beginning and the Context. Thanks are also due to Teariki Mei for his wise counsel. I am especially grateful to Isabelle and Susan Sherrard for agreeing to write a foreword. Their wisdom and experience have helped me to grow.

The decision to publish has brought the welcome support and encouragement of Yvonne Shadbolt and Jocelyn Keith, and the expert assistance of Daphne Brasell Associates Press.

Through it all there has been unfailing love and encouragement from my precious family.

I give my heartfelt thanks to each person who has shared in some way in this seemingly unending, sometimes daunting, mostly exhilarating, always challenging experience.

The nursing fraternity has shown enormous support for the publication of this book. The following list records people and institutions who actively supported this publishing venture by pre-ordering copies. (There were others as well whose names do not appear here.)

Auckland Area Health Board, Auckland Technical Institute Library, Auckland Technical Institute School of Nursing and Midwifery, Liz Brunton, Shona Butterfield, Rachel Cadwallander, Beverly Chappell, Penelope Dunkley, G. M. Eaton – Sx Hospital Trust, Mary Gibbs, Beverly Gummer, Teenah Handiside, Verna Harford, Nola Hatherley, Hamilton Public Library, Amanda Jarvis, Alison Johnston, Jocelyn Keith, Kathryn Kershaw, Merian Litchfield, Catherine Logan, Antoinette McCallin, Margaret McDougall, Grace McGrechan, Helen MacKenzie, Maire McMullen, Manawatu Polytechnic Library, Manukau Polytechnic School of Nursing, Barbara Martin, Judi Anne Mulholland, June Amelia Nasuta, New Zealand Nurses' Association, Greater Wellington Region, New Zealand Nurses' Association Library, Nursing Council of New Zealand, Otago Polytechnic Nursing Department, Yvonne Shadbolt, Isabelle Sherrard, Sally Simms, Southland Polytechnic Library, Annette Stevenson, Taranaki Base Hospital Library, Taranaki Base Hospital Staff Development Unit, Waimate Workplace Committee, Wellington Polytechnic Library, Wellington Polytechnic School of Nursing and Health Education, Wellington Public Library, Gay Williams, Daphne Widdowson.

programmes to prepare nurses for the changed working environment, the author had been keenly aware of this deficiency in nursing's proven body of knowledge. If it was to be corrected, fundamental questions had to be addressed. What is, could be, or should be the role of the newly registered nurse in a setting where nursing care is primarily given by registered nurses? What do students need to learn – about themselves, about patients, about nursing, about the nursing role and about health and illness?

During this same period there was anxiety within the nursing profession about the high mobility and low retention rate of staff nurses at a time when, because of the new staffing pattern, they were required in increased numbers. Perhaps resolution of this problem could be assisted by a better understanding of the nature of nursing in action. Hopefully, the resulting knowledge could then be used to enhance the status of hands-on nursing, increase the job satisfaction of registered nurses and encourage them to remain in practice.

Reflections on personal nursing experiences also had a major influence on the development of the original research study. Many situations were recalled where nurses had seemed unable to move beyond their preoccupation with tasks and see what was happening to a patient and see what nursing, through them, could offer. Two examples illustrate this.

The first had occurred during a previous field study. Two nurses, one shortly after the other, approached a patient who had recently experienced an abortion at about 16 weeks' gestation. Standing some distance from the patient, both asked the question, 'Are you okay?' After receiving a nod from the patient, both left the room. However, concern for her pallor and air of apprehension led the researcher, taking on the role of nurse, to approach the patient for a closer look. Her pulse was high, her blood pressure low. On lifting the bedclothes, the researcher discovered a large pool of fresh blood coming from the vagina. The patient admitted she did not feel well at all. When asked why she had not said anything to the nurses she replied, 'I didn't like to bother them. They're so busy.' Action by the researcher led to immediate medical intervention and the patient was taken to the operating theatre within a few minutes. In this situation the patient seemed to consider the nurses' apparent 'busyness' to be more important than her own needs. At the same time the nurses were failing to use their nursing wisdom as they approached the patient. Thus, they didn't see the evidence that all

LIST OF TABLES

was not well, in spite of the lack of congruence between the patient's words and behaviour. Why was this so?

The second example came from an experience when the author was working in a surgical ward during a period of 'refreshment' away from her teaching role. She was assigned a patient who was considered a 'problem' and a cause of concern to the charge nurse. Examination of the nursing documentation revealed that no patient problems had been entered on the care plan, while the nursing notes only mentioned that the elderly woman was incontinent and 'seems upset'. She was ready for discharge after surgery for a perforated gastric ulcer. Talking with this elderly woman, and observing her and her behaviour while giving assistance with daily hygiene, led to the identification of a significant number of problems which were amenable to nursing action. Discussion with the patient confirmed the following problems: grief over the death of her only sister four weeks before in a geriatric hospital; guilt that she had not visited her sister in the week before she died; no living relatives; loneliness; fear of going home to a large house where she felt afraid; incontinence at night; deafness; constipation; uncertainty on her feet; painful neck and shoulder; continuing indigestion and dysphagia; inability to shower/bath and dress herself; broken skin along her thoracic spine; excoriation under both breasts; marked oedema of ankles and feet; painful lower legs with very dry, pigmented and fragile skin; oral thrush; inadequate food intake; and nurses continually putting sugar on her porridge – the only food she enjoyed but which she could not eat with sugar!

Experiences like these caused the researcher real concern. Information which could lead to beneficial nursing action was readily available but the registered nurses were not seeing it. Yet more questions were generated and required answers. How do nurses perceive the patient? How do they perceive their work? How do they decide what nursing the patient requires? Do they value, and respond to, individual differences in patient situations? How can nurses be assisted to approach the patient in a spirit of enquiry with their accumulated nursing knowledge and skills ready for application at every moment?

These questions and subsequent reading focused interest on the patterning of the encounter between nurse and patient. Increasingly, the author found herself unsatisfied by the existing published conceptualisations of nursing. Indeed, questions about what actually happens in the interaction between nurse and patient multiplied and became more fundamental as reflection progressed. Finally, it was decided to undertake a study of nursing in action in an attempt to discover the phenomena that are within the domain of the nurse. In the familiar nursing setting of the surgical ward, data would be gathered from a group of patients and nurses while the former were undergoing planned surgery. The question to be answered was: What is happening here?

The giving and receiving of nursing care during elective surgery is particularly amenable to study as a total process. In contrast to emergency admissions, both patients and nurses can be interviewed before and on admission, during the immediate peri-operative period and during the rehabilitation phase following surgery. Also, the length of time each patient is in hospital is usually predictable and expected to be of short duration. Yet, during this time, the patient's nursing status changes dramatically, passes from independence at admission to total dependence during the surgery, then through the recovery period back to increasing independence as the time for discharge approaches. It is as if this one experience is a microcosm of nursing, as each patient rapidly passes through the full range of patient states which nurses can encounter in any setting.

Another reason for the choice of the surgical ward as the research setting was the medical presence. Stevens asserts that nursing's domain, 'however it is is eventually characterised', is different from that of medicine, and goes on to make the thought-provoking statement

> By this, I do *not* mean that nursing should find its subject matter by ignoring medicine and pretending that it will go away. While I welcome the movement of nursing into well care (it is an area where health needs can effectively be met by nurses), I decry the movement to well care when it is done as a way to avoid contact with medicine and its domain. Simply put, I do not think nursing can afford to abandon the care of the ill – the care of those under medical therapy – in its attempt to establish its own independence. Indeed, I think it is a common misconception to think that nursing decisions that take into account the medical regimen are therefore subservient to medicine. On the contrary, the medical regimen is a critical factor, but only one factor in the nursing decision. Knowing and understanding the medical regimen, in all its implications, is neces-sary but not sufficient knowledge for any nursing decision. (Stevens, 1979, pp 259–260)

Within the surgical ward, and throughout the hospital setting, nursing care often appears to be based primarily on the medical model of care, with its main focus on the diagnosis of a pathological problem and the associated cure-oriented medical intervention. Any definition of nursing which uses this model ascribes to the nurse a primary role of assistant to the medical staff. Consequently, nursing is often perceived to be a subordinate service rather than an independent profession with its own work to perform for and with the patient. Confirmation of nursing's contribution to patient care within the hospital setting is dependent on the generation of research-based models which identify a specific nursing perspective. In this way, the patient's need for nursing, and the nursing response, could be separated from, but interrelated with, the individual's need for medical care.

During the current period of rapid change in the New Zealand health service, when issues related to nursing – the service and its personnel – are constantly under scrutiny, this distinction is of critical importance. If the 'assisting' perspective holds sway, then nursing is devalued and the justification for a qualified nursing work-force is open to argument. One New Zealand nursing leader argued that '. . . specification of a central core of nursing articulated universally and applied consistently may move nursing from a defensive position implicit in the medical model, thereby focusing attention on the nursing role' (Salmon, 1982, p 121).

Another New Zealand nurse has shared her regret that many nurses view the assisting role as the 'crux of their practice' and goes on to point out that such a perspective of practice is often unwitting, whereas '. . . the nurse of quality knows that nursing is an entity of itself, not controlled by other professionals, which must be given due importance and due time to practice' (Nightingale, 1983, p 22).

Unfortunately, although nurses 'of quality' may indeed see nursing as having an independent service to offer to any person whose health and wellness is threatened, the identification of specific nursing dimensions to aid translation of this ideal into practice has proved difficult and elusive. It became apparent that there is a paucity of theoretical research which investigates phenomena as they occur within the challenging arena of nursing practice, particularly when this occurs concurrently with an active medical regime. This observation is supported in the current nursing literature. For example, Kim points out that there has been 'little systematically presented empirical evidence in nursing', and this means that 'theories based on inductive generalisations have not been well developed' (Kim, 1983a, p 178). Similarly, after reviewing 22 reports of studies of adults undergoing elective surgery, Johnson concludes that 'more theoretically oriented research is required before a description of the processes of coping with surgery can be developed' (Johnson, 1984, p 128). She believes that there would be significant value for nursing practice from sound theoretical research in this example of a 'stressful health care experience' (ibid, p 130).

While nursing's development as a profession is enhanced by the development of nursing theory, this only has value when it can be translated into beneficial action for the patient. Although medicine is widely considered to have the major role in the treatment of disease, the multiple dimensions of any illness experience go far beyond the medical scope of practice. If those aspects of the patient's situation which can benefit from nursing can be identified, this would give nurses a mandate for independent action within a specified scope of practice. Such a defined role would not only be of value to the patient but would also complement and facilitate the work of medical and other colleagues.

And so the scene was set for a field study which used a qualitative research method. The outcome (presented in Chapters 2–8) is a 'discussional' grounded theory (Glaser and Strauss, 1967, p 115) – a systematic description of the properties of each of the categories generated from the data. The patient's experience has been conceptualised as a complex social process derived from anthropology – a passage which is worked through in partnership with nursing. In this form, the research outcome is a theoretical framework rather than a developed theory (see Appendix 1).

1   BACKGROUND TO THE NURSING PARTNERSHIP

The research which generated the Nursing Partnership took place in New Zealand at a time of change in nursing education and nursing service within a changing national health service. It was undertaken in a large general hospital which was feeling the impact of these changes. After a century of involvement in the preparation of nurses for registration, the hospital was about to close its three-year general and obstetric nursing programme. Increasing numbers of graduates from the replacement comprehensive nursing programme offered at the local and other technical institutes throughout the country were joining the staff. The proportion of nurses with post-basic nursing qualifications from universities and technical institutes was also increasing.

Nationally, this removal of employee students from the hospital work-force has necessitated the development of new patterns for staffing nursing units. Issues related to the employment and retention of registered nurses in the hospital nursing service have come to the fore, as has the role of the nurse in the new context. Other countries are experiencing, or have experienced, the consequences of similar changes in nursing education. This has also been accompanied by renewed interest in the existing theories of nursing (for example: Johnson, 1968; King, 1971; Levine, 1967; Orem, 1971; Parse, 1981; Roy, 1976; and Rogers, 1970).

All of these issues helped to shape the nursing context in which this study took place. Further discussion, with reference to selected literature, is organised into three sections: The Changing Pattern of Nursing in New Zealand, The Theoretical Basis of Nursing Practice, and The Experience of Hospitalisation.

The Changing Pattern of Nursing in New Zealand

The changes in nursing education since the early 1970s have dramatically altered the nature of the hospital nursing service.

Registered nurses have discovered that their previously predominant role of supervising the work of students has been reduced and replaced by a role as a bedside or hands-on nurse. In this role they become the primary agent for nursing and the model for nursing students. As such, they establish the standard to which these neophyte nurses will aspire after graduation. Two particular aspects of the New Zealand situation have significance for the study and its outcome: the closure of hospital-based nursing programmes, and the role of the registered nurse in an all-qualified work-force.

Closure of Hospital-Based Nursing Programmes

Controversy and change have been, and continue to be, persistent themes in nursing education. Since 1973, the nature of basic nursing education, the type of registration attained, the status of the students, the site of the schools and the conditions of learning have undergone a revolution.

Prior to 1973, a nurse gained registration through one of three types of three-year nursing programmes – general and obstetric, psychiatric or psychopaedic. Schools of nursing were operated by hospital boards which had the primary function of providing a regionally based health service funded by central government. During their training, students were employees of the hospital board, and received wages in return for providing the majority of the bedside nursing in hospitals. Formal education took the form of study days and/or study blocks interspersed with an employment-based rotation through a range of hospital wards.

In 1969, the Review of Hospital and Related Services identified a number of major problems in the existing system of preparing nurses for registration. These included: too many schools; small schools with inadequate learning experiences; inadequate supervision of students on the three nursing shifts; priority given to service needs over the students' learning needs; failure of more than half of the students to complete the nursing programme; a shortage of qualified nurse tutors (Department of Health, 1969, p 41–43).

By the early 1970s, the New Zealand Nurses' Association was seeking government action to transfer nursing education into the system of general education. A major review of nursing education ensued and this, together with concerted action by nurses throughout New Zealand, eventually led to a decision to introduce change (Carpenter, 1971; Department of Education, 1972; New Zealand Nurses' Association, 1973, 1980). On 2 November 1972, the

Minister of Health announced that pilot three-year student-based programmes would commence in 1973 in two technical institutes. After that initial announcement, decisions to increase the number of schools which could offer the new programmes were made on an ad hoc basis annually in the midst of continuing confusion and controversy. In reviewing the impediments to progress in New Zealand nursing, a national workshop reported that the

> . . . continued use of students has served to distort the role of the registered nurse who, once qualified and deemed competent to provide nursing services, tends to become increasingly involved in non-nursing activities . . . but the surest way to ensure that nursing skills are utilised is to remove unqualified persons (students) from the service setting. (Nursing Education and Research Foundation, 1977, p 8)

Finally, at the opening of the Annual Conference of the New Zealand Nurses' Association in 1979, the Minister of Health was able to confirm government commitment to the total transfer of nursing education to technical institutes.

> The transfer . . . is now almost 30% complete. The question which remains is not which way, but at what pace the transition is to proceed. (New Zealand Nurses' Association, 1980, p 11)

Despite this affirmation, the transfer of basic nursing education from hospitals to the general education system was not complete until the mid-1980s. By that time the majority of three-year programmes offered by hospital nursing schools had closed or were closing. Increasing numbers of technical institutes were offering the new integrated three-year programme for registration as a comprehensive nurse.

In these new nursing schools, curricula used the the available conceptual frameworks to provide graduates with the knowledge and skills required for a working life of hands-on nursing. Initially nurse educators combined wisdom borne of experience with creativity until the new curricula could be confirmed or rejected by systematic study. It was expected that nurses would graduate from these new schools with a broad nursing registration which would enable them to exercise the individual responsibility and accountability now required in the nursing service.

As the first class of comprehensive nurses prepared to commence practice, the author, in the role of teacher, described the goal of the programme.

> What we have striven to do is to produce a nurse acceptable in the New Zealand setting, able to adjust to the changing pattern of health care delivery, wanting to continue to give patient care after graduation. (Christensen, 1976, p 24)

Role of the Registered Nurse in an All-Qualified Work-Force

The traditional reliance on employee students to provide much of nursing's work had led to a strongly hierarchical organisation in which nursing was described as a list of tasks and duties. These were distributed among the members of the nursing team according to the present knowledge and skills level of each person. 'Rigid rules and routines [were] established to avoid errors' (Carpenter, 1971, p 18). Supervisory positions abounded. Much of the work of registered nurses involved management of the unit and supervision of unqualified students. Indeed, the author recalls a final-year nursing student in a hospital programme in 1973 stating, 'I don't really want to pass my exams because I won't be allowed to be a nurse any more!'

There was concern over the consequences of a situation whereby patients were being nursed by students during critical life events, and registered nurses were not able to use their considerable knowledge and skills in bedside nursing. The Board of Health concluded that 'professional nursing services should be supplied by those qualified to provide such services' (Board of Health, 1974, p 21). This conclusion had already been reached by many nurses. For example, a member of the Professional Services Committee of the New Zealand Nurses' Association in 1972 had given her support to a qualified nursing service.

> Let the nurse having responsibility for the care of the sick, not be the one under stress of learning the fundamentals of care. Let her be the qualified nurse. Confident that she has been well prepared to practise the skills of this, her chosen career. (Burgess, 1972, p 5)

The advent of a qualified nursing service had considerable implications for nurses and patients. A new front person, the registered nurse, would be at the patient's bedside – nursing. Thus, the staff in most nursing situations would be registered nurses who required limited supervision. This significant change led to 'an upsurge of interest in the methods of delivering nursing care and in the preparation of nurses' (New Zealand Nurses' Association, 1976, p 8).

In preparation for the arrival of new graduates from student-based comprehensive programmes, nurses within the hospital nursing service 'now turned their thinking towards clinical practice' and became 'more and more interested in the quality of the service they provide for their clients' (Pitts, 1980, p 3). A system was required that would encourage the fullest use of the knowledge and skills possessed by each registered nurse in the nursing team. Due attention had to be given to ensure that those nurses who were now to give nursing care would 'have the opportunity for the stimulation and satisfaction that goes with intellectual and professional growth' (Shaw, 1974, p 5). There was concern that nursing knowledge had 'reached a utilitarian plateau' which would impede 'the vital, over-flowing and expansive kind of care that brings delight to both the person requiring the nurse's care and the nurse herself' (Salmon, 1982, p 19).

This reciprocal linking of the degree of delight experienced by the nurses with the degree of vitality in their nursing was timely. However, a 1984 policy statement on nursing education suggested that 'preoccupation with the minutiae of daily work' was still preventing 'a wider, more constructive and effective nursing approach' (New Zealand Nurses' Association, 1984, p 49). Career satisfaction is largely dependent on the way in which nurses view, and are helped to view, their 'daily work'. Therefore, it seems essential that nurses who are about to embark on life as registered nurses have access to at least one research-based theoretical model of nursing which reflects both the potential and the reality of nursing practice. In this way their accumulating nursing knowledge and skill can be put to the best use and continually challenged so that they will experience personal and professional satisfaction in a hands-on nursing role.

Against the background of this dynamic restructuring in New Zealand nursing, there remains a genuine concern that nursing's survival is under threat if its theoretical basis is not enhanced through research.

> [There] exists today an unprecedented need for clarification of the uniqueness of nursing practice, lest over-riding forces in contemporary society lead to the disintegration of nursing as a distinct profession. (Salmon, 1982, p 111)

Such unease at the continuing lack of a sound theoretical basis and at a facilitating practice environment has continued despite the dramatic changes in nursing education and the organisation of the nursing service.

> We have reformed nursing education – taken it out of the hospitals into educational institutions, reduced some of the medical domination, revised and revamped curricula, and sweated over philosophies. All were necessary actions, but I'm not sure they are sufficient conditions for nursing to self-actualise. (Chick, 1983, p 43)

Theoretical Basis of Nursing Practice

In a dramatic account of her own hospitalisation for major surgery, Johnson, a nurse educator and theorist, suggested that nurses should remember that 'our knowledge doesn't necessarily represent the 'whole truth'' (Johnson, 1972, p 133). Even the knowledge base currently available to nurses is considered to lack a 'validated' shape which would identify it as an independent profession (Roberts, 1980). At the present time, there is an urgent need to develop a system of nursing knowledge 'that will increase the percentage of rational and explained acts in the total repertoire of what the nurse does in nursing' (Kim, 1983b, p 119).

Nursing's long history and rich diversity of setting and action leaves little doubt that nursing 'exists', although its theoretical basis is inadequately articulated. This means that practice is derived from experience and tradition rather than from research-based nursing theory.

Further discussion on this point will focus on an examination of three relevant issues: Nursing's Origins in Maternal Nurturance, Nursing as a Situation-Specific Activity, and The Developing Theoretical Basis of Nursing Practice.

Nursing's Origins in Maternal Nurturance

There is a linguistic link between nursing and the act of nourishing that clarifies the nature of nursing. 'The idea of nursing as the suckling of an infant is ancient. Thus, the activity of nursing can be considered as an integral, essential part of human life and development' (Weatherston, 1979, p 366). By the nineteenth century the meaning of nursing had broadened to encompass the activities associated with the maintenance of health among family members and their care in times of illness – activities that were almost exclusively performed by the women of the family. At that time Nightingale found it necessary to write 'some hints' so that 'every woman' would be able to teach herself 'how to nurse' (Nightingale, 1859, p v). However, in this major work she clearly recognised a separate role for a skilled nurse which was distinct from the nursing component within the social role of 'every woman'.

In the first premise to her science of caring in nursing, Watson confirms that nursing arises from the health-related needs of people as they pass through the various developmental phases and circumstances associated with human life in a social group.

> Caring (and nursing) has existed in every society. Every society has had some people who have cared for others. A caring attitude is not transmitted from generation to generation by genes. It is transmitted by the culture of the profession as a unique way of coping with its environment. Nursing has always held a caring stance in regard to other human beings. (Watson, 1979, p 8)

The thread of compassion and care which, with its emphasis on enhancing the well-being of a child or an ill person, has its origins in the general nurturing role of mother, has been retained, through the efforts of Nightingale and many others, as an essential characteristic of nursing today. But separation of the role of nurse from the 'natural' female role has not been easy, with many people still seeming to believe 'that nursing consists of simple tasks which anyone could perform' (Roberts, 1980, p 33).

Isobel Hampton, a prominent nineteenth-century nurse, told nurses at a meeting at the 1893 Chicago World's Fair that

> . . . the idea still prevails in many minds that almost any kind of woman will do to nurse the sick, and that the woman who has made a failure of life in any other way may as a last resource undertake this work. (Hampton 1899/1989, p 124)

Although many have devalued nursing in this way, others have acknowledged the historical context and, furthermore, have suggested that this association with the concept of nurturant caring actually empowers nursing.

> Despite our periodic raillery about the word 'nursing' and the perceived stigma attached to its designation, our occupation is well-named. Nursing is nurturing, nourishing, fostering, caring. Nursing is caring: both the attitude and the activity . . . . Nursing is caring for those who need to be nurtured in relation to their health status, wherever, as long and as frequently as they need it, until that need is removed or revised by recovery, independence or death. (Styles, 1982, p 230)

These characteristics are highly abstract, with both objective and subjective components which are difficult to describe in terminology unique to nursing. Nurse theorists face the problem of distinguishing between the person-to-person caring in both a 'chance kindly act and [a] professional service' (Wiedenbach, 1964, p 20).

Nursing as a Situation-Specific Activity

In the 1950s and 1960s it was common practice for definitions of nursing to focus on the activities undertaken by nurses. Nursing was thought to be definable as a list of what nurses do, and the context in which they were performed was considered irrelevant. An example of this approach was a major study sponsored by the California Nurses' Association in 1953 which identified 439 separate nursing functions. However, in recognition of the rate of change in nursing practice – implementing new procedures, discarding of old ones – the report concluded: 'Some will question whether this effort has been worthwhile . . . whether this information will remain timely enough to be useful' (Simmons and Henderson, 1964, p 229–233).

Lists of disparate activities fail to reflect the reality of nursing as it is selectively applied to individual patient situations. In criticising this approach, Simmons and Henderson regretted the fact that the 'patient appears, for the most part, a passive and background figure, sometimes nearly the forgotten man' (ibid, p 233). It is this functional approach which continues to cause considerable difficulty for nursing. In his defence of the essential nurturing/caring orientation of professional nursing, Pearson argues that this is

> . . . fundamental to human life and growth, and is therefore highly valuable. If this was reflected upon, nurses would fiercely hang on to this basis of their role, and society would see it as being precious and worthy of status . . . . In reality, a belief in the importance of this has been lost by nurses and society. Intimate physical care is seen as 'basic nursing', unskilled, and rejected as lowly by qualified nurses who say that they did not train for three years to bath people. So it is delegated to the untrained auxiliary or nursing student . . . . So, the need for nurturing and intimate care which gives rise to the need for nursing is contradicted and denied. (Pearson, 1988, pp 134–5)

If, instead of focusing only on nursing functions, attention is given to their purpose in relation to a person, there is a critical change in emphasis to involve nurturing/caring for that person as well as exercising nursing judgement in relation to the presenting status of the recipient. And 'there is nothing simple about patients' (ibid, p 141). The dynamic impact of such situation-specific nursing activity is affirmed by Weatherston.

> The nurse who cares for a person paralysed by a stroke, by dressing her and washing her, is not nursing. Nursing would involve helping the person wash and dress herself, if at all possible . . . . Quality of life is valued, thus we help the person regain independence, and help create a sense of well-being. (Weatherston, 1979, p 369)

Such a view of nursing accepts that there are a range of activities which are essential to human living. The assumption is made that the 'normal' human state is independence in the performance of these activities. This self-care ability may be influenced by a multitude of internal and external challenges throughout life. Associated with each activity is a range of performance criteria and a point at which the person requires assistance to accomplish the activity. In her well-known statement on the uniqueness of nursing, Henderson suggests that nursing has a specialised role in decision-making and action related to this aspect of human living.

> [The] unique function of the nurse is to assist the individual, sick or well, in performance of those activities contributing to health or its recovery (or peaceful death) that he/she would perform unaided if he/she had the necessary strength, will or knowledge. And to do this in such a way as to help him/her gain independence as rapidly as possible. (Henderson, 1966, p 15)

This view that nursing focuses on the ability of the patient to fulfil the requirements of daily living is shared by others, including theorists King and Orem.

> The dynamics of nursing can be described as a constant restructuring of relationships between the nurse and the patient to cope with existential problems and to learn ways of adapting or adjusting to changes in daily activities. (King, 1971, p 103)

> Health derived or health related limitations for engagement in continuing care of self or care of dependents is the reason why human beings can benefit from nursing. (Orem, 1978, tape)

With the focus of nursing moving to patients in the context of their circumstances, nursing can be clearly perceived as a relationship. To nurse means to be involved with people (MacQueen, 1974, p 12; Gruendeman, Casterton, Hesterly, Minckley and Shetler, 1973, p 30; Toynbee, 1977, p 121). This relationship is characterised by a mutual sharing in which the nurse uses the 'special knowledge' called nursing to supplement the patient's present ability (MacQueen, 1974, p 18; Stevens, 1979, p 261; Rubin, 1969, p 44).

Therefore, the relationship the nurse establishes with each patient is significant. Indeed, Peplau believes that this association is '. . . often more telling in the outcome of a patient's problem than are many routine technical procedures' (Peplau, 1952, p 6). Because of her belief that the impact of the person of the nurse on the nurse-patient encounter is underestimated, King gave priority to the person-to-person relationship in her theory (King, 1971; 1978).

As a nurse I am one of the most critical variables in that nursing situation and it is time we recognised our critical variability and how we influence the situation. (ibid, 1978, tape)

Kaperick describes nurses as 'people helpers' and goes on to suggest that each nurse has

. . . many tools to work with and yet the most important one is her self. How she uses herself is the key to really helping people. How she lives her life with the patient from the time they are together, be it minutes, hours or days, will determine whether both parties grow as people or whether it was a waste of time. (Kaperick, 1971, p 23)

Such descriptions confirm that the nurse is the effective instrument required to translate nursing into action relevant to each patient's situation. Skill in judgement as well as performance are critical to an optimal nursing outcome.

Outsiders have not traditionally associated 'thinking' with nurses and nursing. 'A good nurse historically has been measured from the neck down: busy hands and busy feet' (Manthey, 1980, p 35). Indeed, the 'good' nurses were ones who could model themselves on the experienced nurses they learned from and perform the 'tasks' of nursing as they saw them performed. Today's 'new emerging culture of nursing' means that 'emphasis is being placed on the creative "thinker" of nursing practice and less emphasis is given to the continuous "doer"' (Leininger, 1970, pp 72–73).

If it is recognised that nurses do make decisions based on an appraisal of people within a specific situation; then theoretically nursing can be confirmed as an independent activity. However, there continues to be difficulty expressing nursing's independence in a way that identifies it as a separate discipline in a collaborative but equal relationship with other health-related disciplines, particularly medicine. 'For any real improvement to occur, the public must make a distinction between what the physician has to offer and what the nurse has to offer' (Ashley, 1976, p 131). It is this close association with medicine, particularly in the hospital setting, which 'has been detrimental in establishing a separate identity for nursing' (Mundinger, 1980, p 8).

Over recent years, more and more procedures for patient management – diagnostic, remedial and monitoring – have become available to hospital-based medical care. While the decision-making to prescribe their use remains in the medical sphere, the performance of many of these procedures has been delegated to nursing. This occurs primarily because of the nurse's continuing presence with the patient in contrast to the intermittency of medical visits. While some have seen the performance of these as enhancing the status of nursing, this development can be viewed as the antithesis of what nursing needs at this time.

> . . . nurses are being encouraged to undertake more and more medically related tasks such as venepuncture, haemoglobin estimation and first assessment visits. To the extent that they enter the domain of diagnosis and assessment, they are increasing their relative subordination, as there can be no equality of knowledge and responsibility in medical decision making . . . . Conversely, to the extent that nurses maintain their focus on nursing care and development of expertise, they move away from subordination to doctors and towards professional independence and autonomy. (McIntosh and Dingwall, 1978, p 123)

Peplau identified nurses' perception of their independence in on-the-spot decision-making as a key issue in the consolidation of nursing as a separate discipline.

> In each situation, the readiness of nurses to think for themselves and to share in the determination of what can be done to meet patient needs, or their readiness to permit others to make all decisions and govern all of their actions, is an important factor in defining nursing and what it can do. (Peplau, 1952, p 16)

While it is not valid to charge either nurses or nursing with intellectual subordination, there is considerable potential for nursing to be perceived as being dependent on medicine. This arises from nursing's poorly defined theoretical base; from the conditions under which nurses have been socialised into the profession; and from the perceived lack of control over their own work experienced by individual nurses. Coser could be speaking of today's surgical ward as well as those of the 1960s when she expresses her belief that the nurse's

> . . . own feeling of freedom to make decisions, along with the new philosophy of self-help inherent in post-operative care, encourages her to let patients make as many little decisions about themselves as physical conditions permit . . . . Independent nurses help make independent patients. (Coser, 1962, p 144)

Developing Theoretical Basis of Nursing Practice

The 1960s and 1970s saw the publication of a number of theoretical models which ascribed nursing-relevant dimensions to the patient. For example, Johnson conceptualised the patient as a behavioural system; Rogers as an energy field; Orem as a self-care agency; and Roy as an adaptive system (Johnson, 1968; Rogers, 1970; Orem, 1971; Roy, 1976). These, and other nursing models of the patient, were attempts to look at the human being in a way which would enable nurses to work out patient states which could benefit by nursing intervention.

The identification of problems associated with a particular theoretical perspective would then allow the nurse to plan actions which could be expected to improve the patient's situation. Nursing could then be viewed as a process. One of the first nurses to speak of the nursing process described it as comprising the interaction of three elements: '(1) the behaviour of the patient, (2) the reaction of the nurse and (3) the nursing actions which are designed for the patient's benefit' (Orlando, 1961, p 36). Gradually, however, steps were assigned to the nursing process which closely linked it with problem-solving activities performed by the nurse, or the scientific method: data gathering; diagnosing; planning; implementing; evaluating (for example, Yura and Walsh, 1973; Zimmerman and Blainey, 1970; Carrieri and Sitzman, 1971; American Nurses' Association, 1973; New Zealand Nurses' Association, 1981).

The linking of a conceptual model of the patient with the problem-solving method known as the nursing process led to an extension in descriptions of nursing. Now there was a way of working out when nursing was needed and a format for translating the interpretation into a planned nursing response. This theoretical control over decision-making in relation to patient care was seen as having the potential for elevating nursing to the status of an independent discipline.

> The nursing process enables a nurse to realise her potential as an independent decision-maker who has command over competencies which heretofore were not used in carrying out predominantly assistance-type functions. (Mauksch and David, 1974, p 3)

When on-the-spot decision-making is seen to be a characteristic component of nursing theory, it requires each nurse to develop a strong personal nursing identity. Nurses are required to maintain the currency of their nursing knowledge and skills so that a valid theoretical basis is provided from which appropriate nursing strategies for individual nursing situations can be selected.

> Judgement is personal in character; it will be exercised by the nurse according to how clearly she envisions the purpose to be served, how available relevant knowledge is to her at the time, and how she reacts to prevailing circumstances such as time, setting and individuals. (Wiedenbach, 1964, p 27)

There is evidence that 'the public image of nursing is gradually changing from the traditional "bed-pan servant" to an intellectual nurse with diverse skills and talents' (Leininger, 1970, p 73). This infusion of a theoretical basis into nursing practice is associated with an increasing recognition that nursing theories need to recognise nursing's concern with the patient's 'immediate present' (Rubin, 1969, p 44; Greene, 1979, p 62; Stevens, 1979, p 262).

> Nursing time is essentially the 'now'. It is the actual moment or period, day or night, when the nurse is in contact with her patient . . . . The nurse's area of responsibility makes her focus not only on the physical immediacy of the patient but also on his immediate conceptions. (Wiedenbach 1964, p 15)

Continuity and immediacy are very difficult ideas to convey in a theory. Some recent attempts at theorising have attempted to meet this challenge by the use of the gerundial form[1] for concepts (Roper, Logan and Tierney, 1980; Parse, 1981). At the Fifth National Conference on Nursing Diagnoses in 1982 Roy reported on a theoretical framework developed by a group of nurse theorists which included nine conceptualised patterns of human functioning using the gerundial form: 'Exchanging; communicating; relating; valuing; choosing; moving; perceiving; knowing; and feeling' (Roy, 1984, p 28).

This present, continuous focus in nursing is consistent with the concept of nursing's purpose as assisting people through the whole of a health-related event by helping them through the many moments which comprise the experience. Nursing requires a theoretical shape that encourages its practitioners to apply the full repertoire of nursing's knowledge and skills in each encounter while remaining sensitive to the patient's total experience.

Experience of Hospitalisation

The hospital can be viewed as a place characterised by the inevitable presence of tension, of role conflict, and of culture clash between the nurse and the patient (Congalton and Najman, 1971; Taylor, 1970). It is also commonly perceived as a place of fear of the known and the unknown, with the consequent distress posing a potential challenge to the health of the person who becomes a patient (Salmond, Powell, Gray and Barrington, 1977, p 45).

If, as suggested by Taylor, 'a hospital is designed to care for sick persons while cures are attempted', then both fear and hope are associated with becoming a patient in hospital (Taylor, 1970, p 7). Paradoxically, there may be circumstances when hospitalisation, and even surgery, are welcomed by the patient.

> Having had to cope with very debilitating symptoms, such as acute gallbladder spasms, the patient is happy to be in the hospital even though he is anxious to some degree. He is grateful that he will soon be relieved of his aggravating symptoms. (Gruendemann et al, 1973, p 13)

Most people still regard it as an experience to be avoided.

> Nobody likes to enter the hospital, even if its going to make him better, and we all know why. Checking into a hospital means putting your trust in strangers, in an alien place. (Gots and Kaufman, 1978, p 1)

Hospital staff and patients necessarily view the hospital from different perspectives. For the hospital staff, it is their place of work 'where the crises of patients and their families form the basis of everyday routines'; for the patient, it may be a matter of life and death (Rosenthal, Marshall, Macpherson and French, 1980, p 13). Indeed, the perspectives are so different that nurses may not find their nursing knowledge of real value if there is a role change and a nurse becomes a patient (Johnson, 1972, p 133).

In the setting for this study, the hospital becomes the patient's temporary home while undergoing surgery. The person has to leave familiar surroundings and withdraw from the full expression of usual social roles. On admission, a number of new relationships, including that of patient to the nursing staff, are entered into, but the upcoming surgery, and thus the role as patient to the surgeon, has pre-eminence. 'In the eyes of the patient all other activities are naturally subordinate to this primary purpose' (White, 1972, p 12).

Despite the primacy of the surgery, and therefore the surgeon, it is possible to argue that admission to hospital is necessitated primarily by the need for nursing care during the medical intervention and its consequences (McClure and Nelson, 1982, p 59). In this view, discharge would then be a consequence of nursing no longer being required, although this decision usually remains clearly in the control of medical staff.

Dependency is a state often associated with the role of hospital patient, particularly when the admission is for surgery. Customary autonomy is temporarily forfeited as the patient recognises a dependence on the expertise of others and 'hands over to other people the right to make decisions about his body' (Levitt, 1975, p 498; Taylor, 1982, p 209). This willingness to relinquish control and trust other persons because of their specialised knowledge is not, according to Remen, an unusual event.

> In times of specific need we frequently choose to trust others whose training and expertise prepare them to act on our behalf better than we might be able to ourselves, given the circumstances. We form many relationships in this way; with lawyers, architects, accountants, electricians and many others, physicians and nurses among them. Forming such relationships is a responsible choice, a legitimate means of acting to get our needs met. (Remen, 1980, p 215)

If it is accepted that this willingness to trust an expert is a common occurrence in a society with a large number of specialised roles, it may be more appropriate to perceive the patient's role as a complex one with co-existing elements of autonomy and dependency. This leads to the possibility that the patient possesses an expertise which counterbalances the patient's dependency on the expertise of others. Such a view is illustrated by the following two quotations – from a nurse and then a doctor.

> The patient is unequal to the nurse in ability to make generalized professional judgements. On the other hand, the patient is also an

expert in something: he is an expert in knowing his own body, his own responses and experiences. He is an expert in the particularization that is himself. (Stevens, 1979, p 260)

Professional and patient bring with them into the setting of illness two different sorts of information which are relevant to the task at hand. Both need to be willing to educate and be educated by the other, as neither can take responsibility for doing his or her part in the recovery of health without the information which the other has. (Remen, 1980, p 216)

In the considerable literature on the role of the patient in hospital, a valuable insight is gained from the personal reflections of people who have been recently in the role. One nurse spoke of the difficulty she experienced in becoming a patient and revealed that she had even found herself withholding significant information, particularly her feelings and reactions, from the staff. Consequently, she did not always get appropriate nursing assistance (Johnson, 1972, p 127). From the experiences of 200 patients, Levitt discovered that 'widespread humour and tolerance' were often facades used to avoid 'such feelings as anxiety, fear or depression' (Levitt, 1975, p 497). In a study of patients who have survived a severe illness, Smith found that the external demeanour of patients may not reflect what is going on inside.

A person who is attractively dressed in robe and slippers, surrounded by flowers and cards, may give the impression of requiring little from the nurses. One can be anxious and lonely among the flowers; one can be ill-informed about self-care though surrounded by greeting cards. (Smith, 1981, p 89)

An insight into how nurses can gain access to the patient's real feelings comes from Johnson's belief that she wanted a nurse with whom she 'felt comfortable' before she would be willing to share herself, even in the presence of troublesome feelings (Johnson, 1972, p 132). A high level of competency in, and appropriate use of, nursing skills is also highly valued by patients and, thus, engenders trust and comfort (ibid, p 132; Taylor, 1970, p 65).

Finally, in a study of the value placed on specific nursing activities by nurse and patients, White found that patients gave priority to skills related to 'personal hygiene and physical comfort', and only valued the nurses' work in the here-and-now circumstances associated with the hospital experience. She concluded that

> . . . for most patients, hospitalisation is but a brief moment in a lifetime . . . . Instead of talking so globally about meeting patients' needs, nurses should concentrate on the things they really can do to make illness in the hospital a more tolerable experience. (White, 1972, p 12)

The literature on the meaning of hospital for patients raises a number of issues relevant to this research study. There are constant reminders that each patient's experience is a personal one and a relevant nursing theoretical perspective must allow for the expression of that perplexing, and challenging, individuality.

> Hospitalisation may be experienced as lonely or boring for some, and busy, interesting and curious for others. It may mean a loss of identity, or a feeling of worth. (Wu, 1973, p 70)

In this chapter, selections from the extensive nursing and related literature have been used to discuss the nursing context of the study. Changes in nursing education and nursing service in New Zealand since 1970, current theoretical concepts about nursing practice, and aspects of the meaning of hospitalisation for the patient have all been described. There is no doubt that both the literature and the author's experience sensitised her to the field before, during and after the study. However, the theoretical outcome emerged from the data even though its links to nursing's heritage are apparent.

---

[1] A noun ending in -ing formed from a verb to indicate a continuous action or state.

2 THE NURSING PARTNERSHIP

The Nursing Partnership offers a new way of looking at what happens when a nurse offers learned expertise to a person who is passing through a health-related experience. Nursing's specialised assistance is needed to help minimise the impact on the person, and family, of a health problem and its associated treatment regimen. This theoretical framework, generated from the reality of nursing as it occurs in one setting, assigns a specific shape to the encounter between nurse and patient. It clarifies the contribution nursing alone can make to optimise each person's experience. In this way it both complements and facilitates the work of medical and other colleagues with whom nurses work. Thus, it serves to revalue nursing in a way that can assist the registered nurse to put to full use available nursing knowledge and skills for the benefit of all concerned, but particularly for the patient and the nurse. Consequently, it has potential value for nursing practice, education and research.

It is important to note that the framework was developed from the data using the inductive strategies associated with the grounded-theory method.[1] The nurses and patients who participated in the study did not know of its existence, but their behaviour provided the cues which eventually led to the conceptualisation of this book's theory. From one perspective, the Nursing Partnership can be considered an idealised vision of nursing as it 'should' be. From another, it is nursing as it 'is'. In this latter preferred view, the partnership and its component elements can be found in the real world of nursing practice, but they lack recognition and integration. Thus, they do not serve to guide nursing practice, although they have the potential to do so.

There are three major interrelated elements within the Nursing Partnership: Passage, Mutual Work, and Context. Each will be briefly discussed before the detailed model is presented and each concept defined.

25

Passage

Passage is a social process which can be used to describe an experience of significant change in a person's circumstances. In his classic description of rites of passage, van Gennep likened the life of an individual within society to the pattern of the universe.

> The universe itself is governed by a periodicity which has repercussions on human life, with stages and transitions, movements forward, and periods of relative inactivity . . . . For groups as well as individuals, life itself means to separate and to be reunited, to change form and condition, to die and to be reborn, to wait and to rest, and then to begin acting again, but in a different way. (van Gennep, 1960, pp 3, 189)

From this perspective, life is viewed as a 'series of passages' from one age group to another, from one social status to another, from one place to another, and so on (ibid, p 2). Writing in the first decade of this century, van Gennep, a Flemish anthropologist, proposed the concept of passage in a theoretical interpretation of initiation ceremonies, such as puberty and marriage, within indigenous communities. However, the concept of passage can be broadened to include other critical life experiences. Glaser and Strauss, sociologists, applied the concept of passage to a number of life events described in the research literature, including having tuberculosis and poliomyelitis, recovery from illness, going through medical school, and being a mental patient (Glaser and Strauss, 1971, pp 6–7). Their own research among dying patients generated a passage of dying (Glaser and Strauss, 1968).

The association of passage with a particular experience of change through time has been used recently by another nurse. Parker has conceptualised the pathway of patients with leukaemia as the 'cancer passage' (Parker, 1985, pp 96–119). This passage seeks to portray the patient's illness in the context of a total life situation rather than focusing on a process with distinctive nursing dimensions which includes a framework for nurse-patient collaboration.

Recently, the closely related concept of transition has been used by two nurses to describe experiences of 'passage from one life phase, condition or status to another' (Chick and Meleis, 1986, p 238). They suggest that each transition has at least three phases: entry, passage and exit (ibid, p 240). Although written from a different perspective, as a content analysis of the concept of transition as it has relevance for nursing, their paper encouraged the author to conceptualise passage as it had emerged from this research.

> Nursing practice based on a transition model would run counter to therapeutic interventions aimed only at cure. Return to a disease-free state may not be possible, and even the premorbid level of health may be unattainable. A goal for nursing is that the client emerge from any nursing encounter not only more comfortable and better able to deal with the present health problem, but also better equipped to protect and promote self health for the future. (ibid, p 244)

As conceptualised in the Nursing Partnership, a person embarks on a passage which is characterised by the giving and receiving of nursing in order for the person, as patient, to make optimal progress through a health-related experience such as surgery. Within this passage the patient is the passagee – the person who is undergoing the experience – and the nurse is the agent – the instrument through which nursing is translated into action.

A patient lives through any life experience as a whole and, thus, each of the coexisting passages in which a person is involved has an impact on, and is affected by, all other concurrent passages. For example, the person's life stage passage, such as growing old or adolescence, will have a significant impact on the nature of the passage through nursing care in partnership with the nurse.

In addition, patients differ with respect to the internal and external conditions which exist during a passage. They also vary in the life experiences which have preceded this particular passage, and the resources they have built up during their lifetime to manage such challenging events. Thus, while the overall pattern of a passage through the Nursing Partnership exists for all patients, the situational reality is variable and may or may not lead to a beneficial passage.

The actions of the medical staff – in this case the surgery and its medical management – have a major influence on the shape of the Nursing Partnership because of the ongoing effect they have on the patient. Indeed, it is the intervention by medical personnel and its aftermath that cause the patient to need nursing. Within the partnership itself there is a matrix of interrelated activities which are significant to one another and to the patient's passage as a whole. Changes in any aspect of the patient's circumstances have an impact on the total experience, and the nature of the Nursing Partnership.

The patient's passage through the Nursing Partnership has a strong temporal dimension with a definable beginning and end. It actually commences before that person's admission to hospital with the prelude experience which is conceptualised as the Beginning. After admission, when the nurse and patient meet each other for the first time, three stages or phases have been identified: Entering the Nursing Partnership or Settling In — a period of transition characterised by separation from the 'old' and incorporation into the 'new'; Negotiating the Nursing Partnership — the ongoing process during which patient and nurse work together to cushion the impact on the patient of the disturbances associated with hospitalisation and surgery; and Leaving the Nursing Partnership or Going Home — the period of transition from the now familiar 'new', being a patient, back to the 'old', the changed home situation incorporating the impact and continuing effects of the surgery. The negotiating phase coexists with both of the other phases. The exact times for the completion of Settling In and the commencement of Going Home are not specified, but the changed behaviour of nurse and patient confirms the presence of each phase.

There is no simple linear progression through these phases. Instead, there is a recognition that the patient progressing through the Nursing Partnership is involved in a very complex process.

Mutual Work

Within the Nursing Partnership there is a patterned interaction between patient and nurse which is essential to the outcome of the patient's passage. Each participant, that is the patient as passagee and the nurse as agent of nursing, has a specific pattern of work to perform to progress the patient through the experience. For the patient, this work derives from a need to survive the ordeal caused by the problem, entry into hospital and the surgery. By contrast, the work of the nurse is shaped by the nature of nursing and the ability of individual nurses to select appropriate nursing strategies to ease the path of the patient through the passage. Thus, the relationship between the agent and the passagee is unidirectional with the work of both focusing on the patient.

Success in accomplishing this work is not guaranteed. However, the theory has not been developed to the stage where propositional statements can be made to link the work of the nurse with that of the patient and the outcome of the partnership. At this point, only the patterns of work within the immediacy of the patient's ongoing passage during the various phases of the Nursing Partnership have been defined.

Each Nursing Partnership is made up of a number of nursing episodes – encounters between nurse and patient within the immediacy of the patient's situation. Every nursing episode becomes an integral part of the whole social process, building on what has gone before and influencing what is yet to come. The pre-eminence given to situational encounters between nurse and patient as the building blocks of the passage is supported by Benner's recent work on levels of competency in nursing practice (Benner, 1984). She speaks of the expert nurse maximally applying her accumulated wisdom in moments of 'meaningful engagement' with the patient (ibid, p 215). These nurses 'know how to function in the face of unpredictable situations and to adjust their plans to the contingencies of the situation' while remaining constantly aware of the place this moment has in the patient's total experience. (ibid, pp 115, 141).

Watson also offers support for this revaluing of the individual nursing episode when she speaks of the significance of 'caring occasions' in which the nurse and patient are in contact.

> The actual caring occasion in a presenting moment has the potential to influence both the nurse and the patient in the future. The caring occasion then becomes a part of the subjective, lived reality and the life history of both. (Watson, 1985a, p 61)

Within the Nursing Partnership the focus is clearly on the immediacy of the patient's situation throughout the ongoing passage – whatever that might be, whoever else is involved, whatever concurrent passages occur. The gerundial form is used to portray nursing's work as a range of conceptualised activities, all of which are constantly ready to respond to any aspect of the immediate situation as the patient works to make progress through the passage. Thus, both the expression and the goal of each aspect of nursing work are constantly and dynamically changing as nursing outcomes 'are achieved over and over again, in the ongoing immediacy' of the patient's experience (Stevens, 1979, p 264).

Nursing is continually shaping and reshaping in response to the complexities inherent in the present and ongoing circumstances of each patient's passage. This process has been likened to that of an artist at work.

> Much of artistry lies in the skillful application of general principles to specific situations . . . . While general principles can be formulated to help the nurse diagnose and care for patient needs, the effective application of general principles to a specific situation will always depend to some degree on the skill of the individual nurse. (Woolridge, Leonard and Skipper, 1983, p 22)

Nurses who choose to use the Nursing Partnership as the theoretical framework to guide their practice would enter each encounter already thoroughly familiar with the model and with two key questions in mind: What is happening here to the patient at this point in the passage? What can I, as nurse, do to beneficially progress the patient through the passage at this time? At all times the nurse is aware of the need to consider the two linked temporal dimensions – the immediate moment and the ongoing passage.

The need for both parties to work together is essential in order to gain the best possible outcome from the patient's path through the passage. However, clarification of the shape of this mutual work is required.

At the conclusion of her presentation on collaborative decision-making at a recent conference, Kim posed the question: 'If we let the patient know as much as ourselves, why do we need the nurse?' (Kim, 1987, tape). Put another way the question could be: is self-nursing, as distinct from self-care, possible? Within the hypothesised partnership the answer to this question is no. Rather, the nature of patient and nurse decisions and goals within this working relationship arise from the distinctive expertise each requires to perform their own specific work to achieve an optimal outcome for the patient. Thus, while the patient's wisdom is recognised and valued, nursing wisdom remains with nurses as they give specialised assistance to support the patient through the passage. For example, self-care in all, or at least some, aspects of daily living is a common goal of patient's work, and encouraging that self-care potential for the patient's immediate and ongoing situation by the use of nursing strategies is the related nursing goal.

While this need to work together is essential, there is a significant lack of balance in this relationship between nurse and patient during the Nursing Partnership. This is reflected in the different language used to describe each participant's pattern of work. The patient's work focuses on self and the personal dimensions of the ongoing passage. Thus the focus of each activity is stated, for example, interpreting the experience, managing self. However,

continuous passage. Although thei[r]
patients and nurses view nursing as a [
finding is consistent with Watson's s[
an integrated objective/subjective co[
the 'meaning that nursing may have [
and allows 'the nursing presence to exi[
the nurse is not present physically' (V[
case, the objective component is th[
patient contact, and the subjective co[
of continuity expressed by patients an[

Anonymous Intimacy, the second [
reality of the patient's relationship w[
hours of the nursing day within a hospi[
action by a number of nurses within m[
nurses contribute to a single patient's [
usually have contact with many patie[
relationships between patient and nurse[
theoretical interpretation which clair[
acknowledge the existence of some degr[
the midst of the very personal, often [
nursing. Nurses have access to an [
patients because of the nature of their w[
patient and nurse know each other well [

If nursing is a partnership in whi[
personal anonymity and interchangeabili[
each patient's passage is shared among t[
contact with that individual. Thus, it [
single nurse to regard the patient as 'n[
worthwhile, even essential, to acknowle[
role in a particular patient's overall passa[
and support each individual nurse's res[
decision-making within every nursing [
would be different from that of the pri[
involves the 'allocation and acceptance o[
for decision-making to one individual' [
Consequently, the nurse assigned to the [
shift is required to perform the 'care task[
nurse (ibid, p 34).

Mutual Benevolence, the third de[
goodwill between nursing and its recipien[
instances when a patient and a nurse, as hu[

there is an inherent openness in nursing's work, for example, in attending, enabling, appraising. In each nursing episode nurses adjust the focus of their altruistic work to the patient's presenting circumstances.

In her description of the caring relationship between the two parties, Watson also recognises this unidirectional element.

> . . . a patient's personal involvement in a professional relationship . . . is directed toward the problem at hand and its effect upon his or her life. The concern is unavoidably self-directed. In contrast, the personal involvement of the nurse/person is directed away from one's own self and towards the other's self . . . . A professional relationship may and does allow for the nurse person to benefit and be influenced by the other; however, the nurse does not depend upon receiving from the patient to maintain the involvement. (Watson, 1985a, p 65)

While most theoretical models ascribe work of some kind to the nurse, not all come up with the concept of a working patient. There is little doubt that 'many nurses continue to view patients as recipients of care rather than participants in care. "Doing for" or "to" rather than "working with" is a more comfortable position for these nurses' (Rosenthal, Marshall, Macpherson and French, 1980, p 138). However, the Nursing Partnership requires the nurse to view nursing as a collaboration. It sees the nurse 'as a partner in practice with the client rather than a director of practice to, for or at the client' (Pearson and Vaughan, 1986, p 39).

Strauss and colleagues agree with the idea of an actively working patient when they state that 'an observant person can see hospitalised patients working' (Strauss, Corbin, Fagerhaugh, Glaser, Maines, Suczek and Wiener, 1984, p 127). Further support for a conceptualisation that recognises two fully involved participants is given by Berry and Metcalf who have identified the key variant between nursing models of care as the activity/passivity status of the patient (Berry and Metcalf, 1986, pp 596–597). In her work on collaborative decision-making, Kim assumes that 'clients have the resources to be active participants' in their care and to influence, as distinct from make, nursing decisions (Kim, 1983b, p 271).

However, Miller argues that it is theorists, divorced from practice, who 'advocate the active involvement of patients in their own care' while 'practitioners are often employed in an area where cure rather than care is the dominant orientation, and where

patients are seen as passive recipients of
ventions' (Miller, 1985, p 421). This
patient is not reality as it was revealed in
book is based. Patients could be seen to
when this was not recognised by the nurse
this work is to deny reality. Thus, concept
consistent with what is actually happen
'impractical' theoretical notion.

Every nurse-patient episode within t
viewed as being 'always more complex th
standard helping procedures imply' (Kits
patient works through the passage, the nu
nursing work to the pattern of the patient'
time. Not all nursing action will have a
patient's passage. Although nursing wisd
may fail to select and/or perform the nursin
progress a patient to their greatest benefit

It is in the interests of all concer
complete each passage through the Nursin
and effectively as possible within the circu
Responsibility for that is inevitably shared
is a collaborative endeavour between people
gers brought together for a single purpo
their collaboration is dependent on the out
processes in which nurse and patient are i
passage unfolds.

Context

Three specific contextual determinants withi
were discovered during analysis of the fie
while adding to the complexity of the emer
work, served to increase the 'fit' between th
the reality of the giving and receiving of nu
in the data. They influence the nature of t
experienced by both patient and nurse.

The first, Episodic Continuity, is a key
impact on the nature of the nurse-patient
experience of being nursed is viewed as a pa
integration of separate nursing episodes int
experience reflects the continuity associated
Thus, individual nursing episodes become th

along. However, this is not the norm. For the patient, the nurse is a
buffer, a present source of help, a companion through an ordeal.
This service is usually valued and the nurse who provides it is also
regarded with kindness and gratitude. For the nurse, benevolence
is a major characteristic of an altruistically motivated profession in
which specialised knowledge and skill are intertwined with
compassion. Such a perspective seems incompatible with a power
relationship in which one partner seeks to dominate. Benner feared
this could be the case at this time because nursing is influenced by
the prevailing social attitudes where 'power, status, and control are
taken for granted as the basic motivating forces in human inter-
actions', but her investigation 'found nurses who were skilled in
avoiding power plays with their patients' (Benner, 1984, p 48).

The model of the Nursing Partnership presented in Table 1
shows the centrality of the interrelated elements of passage, mutual
work, and context.

As described, this theoretical framework recognises, emphasises and values the 'wonderful and frustrating complexity' of people
in social situations (Mundinger, 1980, p 197). Similarly, it offers
one answer to Watson's desire for the development through qualitative research of 'knowledge about the lived world of human
experience' (Watson, 1985a, p 2).

A brief introduction to each of the concepts within the five
parts of the grounded theory will be presented in sequence: the
Beginning, Settling In, Negotiating, Going Home, and the Contextual Determinants. Although these concepts may be confusing
in isolation from the data, the purpose of this overview is to set the
scene for Chapters 3-8.

The Beginning

The Beginning is the patient's experience with a health-related
problem from initial awareness to admission to hospital for surgery.
Its duration may be anything from days, perhaps even hours, to
years.

This period precedes entry into the Nursing Partnership. In it
the patient adapts to the changed situation and prepares for the
upcoming experience. Three theoretical constructs were developed
from the field data to identify the work during this initial experience which is relevant to nursing: Surfacing the Problem, Preparing
for Intervention, and Interpreting the Experience.

TABLE 1: The Nursing Partnership (Original)

The Work of the Patient

Surfacing the Problem	Becoming a Patient	Managing Self — Centring on Self, Harnessing Resources, Maintaining Equanimity	Maximising Readiness
Preparing for Intervention	Suspending Social Roles	Affiliating with Experts — Acquiescing to Expertise, Fitting In, Retaining Autonomy	Making Arrangements
Interpreting the Experience	Revealing Self	Surviving the Ordeal — Enduring Hardship, Tolerating Uncertainty, Possessing Hope	Discovering Requisites
		Interpreting the Experience — Monitoring Events, Developing Expertise	Resuming Control

The Work of the Nurse

The Beginning	Settling In	Negotiating the Partnership	Going Home
	Admitting	Attending — Being Present, Ministering, Listening, Comforting	Appraising
	Appraising	Enabling — Coaching, Conserving, Extending, Harmonising, Encouraging	Supplementing
		Interpreting, Responding, Anticipating	

Contextual Determinants

Episodic Continuity
Anonymous Intimacy
Mutual Benevolence

Surfacing the Problem

This is the process in which the patient acknowledges the existence of a problem, adapts to the presence of the problem, makes a decision to seek medical assistance, undergoes an experience of diagnosis and testing, receives information on the medical diagnosis, and, finally, accepts the recommendation that surgical intervention is required.

Four different patterns relevant to this process could be identified in the data:

Evolution – the gradual development of a problem, which is not life-threatening, to the stage where non-urgent surgery is the recommended intervention to alleviate its effects;

Crisis on Evolution – the development of a long-standing problem to a critical state which is now potentially life-threatening and urgent surgical intervention has become necessary;

Anticipated Crisis on Evolution – the evolution of a problem to a stage where urgent surgical intervention is required to reduce the risk of either sudden death or fear-inducing debility; and

Crisis – the sudden presentation of a proven or possible malignancy, associated with pain, suffering and death, which requires urgent surgical intervention.

Preparing for Intervention

The patient takes steps to get ready to enter hospital and seeks to become equipped with the resources to withstand the consequences of the problem and the impending surgery.

Interpreting the Experience

Throughout experience with the problem, a patient analyses events as they occur and synthesises them into a meaningful whole. From this whole a selection of details is extracted which the patient forms a personalised account of events.

The Beginning is presented in more detailed form, with illustrations from the field data, in Chapter 3.

Settling In

Settling In is the transition experience in which the patient enters hospital and comes into contact with nursing. Both patient and nurse have their own pattern of work to perform during this phase. This work is summarised in Table 2.

TABLE 2: Settling In

The Work of the Patient

Becoming a Patient
Suspending Social Roles
Revealing Self

The Work of the Nurse

Admitting
Appraising

The Work of the Patient

On admission to hospital for surgery the patient has a range of Settling In tasks to perform. Through this work the patient, supported by the work of the nurse, becomes a patient to the institution, to the medical staff and other health groups within the hospital as well as becoming a partner within the Nursing Partnership.

Three separate but interrelated patterns were developed from the data to explain the work of the patient upon settling in: Becoming a Patient, Suspending Social Roles, and Revealing Self.

Becoming a Patient

The person takes action to make the transition into the patient role. This process is assisted by learning experiences at the time of admission, the person's previous experience(s) of being a patient, and the help of the nurse.

Suspending Social Roles

As the patient moves from home to the hospital, the usual range of social roles and responsibilities are laid aside for the period of hospitalisation and recovery.

Revealing Self

On admission, the new patient is required to become exposed, in word and body, to others, especially nurses and medical staff, and to

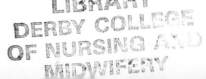

accept the performance of intrusive procedures by people who are virtual strangers.

The Work of the Nurse

The nurse has two major tasks to perform during Settling In: Admitting and Appraising.

Admitting

The nurse undertakes a routine set of tasks on behalf of others – hospital administration, medical staff, and other hospital services – to admit the patient to hospital. Although these are delegated functions, they are given a nursing perspective and have become an integral part of the work of the nurse.

Appraising

Specific activities are initiated by the nurse to establish an information base which will be relevant to nursing the particular patient, and will guide decision-making throughout the partnership.

A discussion on Settling In is presented in Chapter 4.

Negotiating the Nursing Partnership

The major work of nurse-patient negotiation commences at the time of admission to hospital and continues until the patient goes home. It co-exists with, and supports, the work associated with Settling In and Going Home.

Nurse-patient collaboration is required to help the patient proceed through the passage as effectively as possible. It is a dramatic moment-by-moment process as the patient faces the dynamic internal and external challenges which must be continually confronted while in hospital. During this time patient and nurse each undertake their own complex range of activities. These are listed in Table 3.

There is no one-to-one link between the various activities which comprise the work of nurse and patient. The work of both is an integrated matrix in which each individual activity affects the whole. In each nursing encounter the nurse selects from the full range of work strategies the most appropriate combination of actions to assist the patient to progress through the passage.

TABLE 3: Negotiating the Nursing Partnership

The Work of the Patient

Managing Self	Affiliating with Experts
Centring on Self	Acquiescing to Expertise
Harnessing Resources	Fitting In
Maintaining Equanimity	Retaining Autonomy
Surviving the Ordeal	Interpreting the Experience
Enduring Hardship	Monitoring Events
Tolerating Uncertainty	Developing Expertise
Possessing Hope	

The Work of the Nurse

Attending	Enabling
Being Present	Coaching
Ministering	Conserving
Listening	Extending
Comforting	Harmonising
	Encouraging

Interpreting

Responding

Anticipating

The Work of the Patient

The work the patient seeks to accomplish during the passage arises from the total situation. The work is assigned as within the Nursing Partnership because nursing has strategies, which are exclusive to nursing or are shared with other members of the health team, which assist the patient with this work.

Four constructs were generated from the data to describe the major areas in the patient's work which are associated with negotiating the Nursing Partnership: Managing Self, Surviving the Ordeal, Affiliating with Experts, and Interpreting the Experience. Each one has a number of subconcepts.

Managing Self

The patient uses self-management strategies learned since childhood to prepare for and/or endure the experience of hospitalisation and surgery. This work has three identifiable subconcepts:

Centring on Self – the focus on self which permits the patient to maximise the available energy on getting through the experience;

Harnessing Resources – the patient's efforts to control the situation through the use of learned self-management strategies; and

Maintaining Equanimity – the patient's work of striving to attain a personal state of composure, serenity and quietude within, and involves the perceived need to present an acceptable face to others.

Affiliating with Experts

In the hospital a patient receives specialised assistance from a number of experts. In order to get maximum benefit from this, the patient has to learn strategies for interacting with health personnel. Three subconcepts clarify this task:

Acquiescing to Expertise – the selective submission to the experts on whose specialised skill and knowledge the patient is now dependent;

Fitting In – the willingness, and ability, of the patient to adapt to the routines and practices associated with being a hospitalised patient; and

Retaining Autonomy – the patient's selective retention of independence in thought and action while receiving care from experts.

Surviving the Ordeal

The patient undertakes work aimed at enduring the various experiences associated with hospitalisation and the surgery itself. Three subconcepts expand this aspect of the work:

Enduring Hardship – the efforts made by the patient to withstand such experiences as pain, discomfort and inconvenience;

Tolerating Uncertainty – the actions taken by the patient to cope with the lack of certainty about the nature of the problem and the outcome of the surgery, for example, as well as the lack of specialised knowledge which limits decision-making concerning self and circumstances; and

Possessing Hope – the patient's ability to anticipate a future in which there is an improvement in his or her condition and/or circumstances, which may be minutes, hours, days or even weeks away.

Interpreting the Experience

This continues the patient's work, commenced with the Beginning, where events are analysed as they occur and are made into a whole which is personally meaningful. In addition to the constant processing of experiences and information, the patient begins to use an increasing body of knowledge. This is reflected in two additional dimensions in the work:

Monitoring Events – the patient uses increasing knowledge to form opinions on self progress, the work of staff and occurrences in the environment; and

Developing Expertise – the patient progressively processes information and becomes increasingly wise about the situation.

The patient's work is discussed in more detail in Chapter 5.

The Work of the Nurse

The negotiating work of the nurse is dynamic and sensitive as nursing strategies are selectively used to ease the path of each patient through an individual passage. Each action may encompass more than one type of nursing work in the way it is used for a particular patient in a single nursing encounter.

From the data, five theoretical constructs were developed to specify different aspects of nursing work: Attending, Enabling, Interpreting, Responding, and Anticipating.

Attending

Nursing work takes place during the moments of contact between nurse and patient as, in a sense, the nurse accompanies a person through the experience of hospitalisation. Thus, Attending denotes the first essential work of the nurse – being there for the patient. It has four subconcepts:

Being Present – the work of spending time with the patient in order to nurse him or her in the immediacy of the ongoing passage;

Ministering – the selective application of nursing knowledge and skills to meet the identified needs of the patient;

Listening – the nurse's work of concentrating on what the patient is saying and taking heed of this; and

Comforting – the effort made by the nurse to soothe, ease the discomfort, and induce a state of well-being in the patient.

Enabling

This encompasses the nurse's work whereby the patient is assisted to attain the means, opportunity and ability to act within the present circumstances. Five different subconcepts were identified within this construct:

Coaching – the guiding, motivating and teaching work of the nurse;

Conserving – the actions of the nurse which assist the patient to protect, preserve and carefully manage the resources available;

Extending – nursing's work in helping the patient to extend the scope of activities relevant to the current situation;

Harmonising – nursing activity to help attain and/or maintain a beneficial state of synchrony within the patient or between the patient and the environment; and

Encouraging – actions taken by the nurse to inspire the patient with the confidence and the courage to hope, to take action, to make decisions, to accept help.

Interpreting

The nurse uses a number of intellectual activities to continually attach meaning to the status of the patient and the situation. These include observing, monitoring, analysing, translating, contextualising, synthesising and decision-making. Interpreting exists as a separate planned activity as well as being an integral part of every nursing action.

Responding

Throughout the passage the nurse is ready to respond to a perceived change in the patient or the circumstances. This work includes the incidental responding which occurs within each nursing episode as well as a planned, longer-term nursing response.

Anticipating

The nurse is constantly challenged to use both knowledge and previous experience in order to visualise the patient's immediate and/or longer term future and initiate nursing activities to forestall a negative situation and/or facilitate a beneficial outcome.

The nurse's work is presented in more detail in Chapter 6.

Going Home

As the patient's passage progresses, both partners undertake new work specifically associated with preparing the patient for the transition from hospital and from the Nursing Partnership. Time is a significant variable in this phase. An intrinsic sense of healing and progress triggers the patient to begin the preparation for going home. The final decision on the actual time for leaving hospital is usually made by the medical staff, often in consultation with nurses. However, this may not be confirmed until the actual day of discharge. Thus, both patient and nurse may have little time to complete their work if it is delayed until the actual time of discharge is confirmed.

The work of patient and nurse during the final phase of the Nursing Partnership is summarised in Table 4.

TABLE 4: Going Home

The Work of the Patient

Maximising Readiness
Making Arrangements
Discovering Requisites
Resuming Control

The Work of the Nurse

Appraising
Supplementing

The Work of the Patient

The patient engages in a number of tasks in preparation for the transition from hospital or health-care agency to home. There are four separate but interrelated aspects to this work: Maximising

Readiness, Making Arrangements, Discovering Requisites, and Resuming Control.

Maximising Readiness

The patient gets ready as far as possible, in action and thought, to leave the health-care agency and return home as soon as the time and day are confirmed.

Making Arrangements

Prior to going home, the patient takes steps to prepare family and/ or close friends for the return home, and to make appropriate plans for actually going home as soon as the decision is made.

Discovering Requisites

The patient must find out what measures are prescribed by medical and other staff to facilitate a continued recovery at home.

Resuming Control

As the partnership draws to an end, the patient resumes as much self-care as possible after sharing this control with a number of experts while in a health-care agency.

The Work of the Nurse

During the Going Home phase, the nurse seeks, by specific strategies, to make the patient's transition out of the Nursing Partnership as smooth as possible. Nursing is particularly concerned to ensure that the person is as ready as possible to leave the hospital or health-care agency and to manage self-care, or receive appropriate assistance, on returning home. Two concepts were developed from the data to reflect the different aspects of the nurse's work at this time: Appraising and Supplementing.

Appraising

The nurse establishes the patient's potential for self-care after leaving hospital and identifies areas where immediate and longer-term support will be required.

Supplementing

Nursing actions are undertaken to specifically supplement assistance as the patient prepares to leave hospital. Arrangements are also made for specific assistance from nursing and other community services when the patient goes home if nursing judgement indicates this is a necessary adjunct to self- and family-care. Going Home is presented with selected excerpts from the data in Chapter 7.

The Contextual Determinants

The Contextual Determinants are those factors within the nursing context itself which exert a specific influence on the shape of the Nursing Partnership. Three determinants have been identified: Episodic Continuity, Anonymous Intimacy, and Mutual Benevolence.

Episodic Continuity

This is the paradox in which nursing is perceived by both the nurse and the patient as being continuous although it is actually episodic in nature. On examination, nursing is revealed as a series of episodes in which the nurse and patient come into contact for only short periods of time – usually minutes or even seconds – for a specific purpose.

Anonymous Intimacy

In this second paradox, nursing is characterised by a degree of sanctioned closeness despite the fact that patients are usually nursed by a constantly changing group of nurses, and nurses are faced with an ever-changing group of patients as passages are completed and new ones commence.

Mutual Benevolence

This construct refers to the reciprocal goodwill with which both patient and nurse enter the Nursing Partnership, and which each seeks to maintain throughout the relationship.

These Contextual Determinants are further developed in a theoretical discussion, illustrated by excerpts from the field data, in Chapter 8.

This overview of the Nursing Partnership has been brief and presented without support from the rich data which generated the framework. In Chapters 3–8 anecdotes will link each concept to the reality of the practice setting.

1   See Appendix 1 for a discussion on the research method and protocol.

3 THE BEGINNING

For the person involved, admission to hospital for planned surgery continues an individual drama which began years, months, weeks or days ago. Eventually, it has culminated in the person making preparations to enter hospital following the surgeon's recommendation that surgery be performed. There is a complex matrix of actions, reactions and meanings which, in their specific details, are unique to each person's situation. However, it is possible to distinguish patterns which collectively mark the beginning of the person's passage through the Nursing Partnership.

What happens during this prelude to admission is significant for the shape of the developing passage. Each of the concepts within this initial phase may help to form a protocol for nursing appraisal during the Settling In phase. In the discussion which follows, emphasis is given to aspects of this experience which are considered to have an impact on that person's subsequent performance, or work, as a patient.[1]

The Beginning[2]

The moment when a person acknowledges any sign or symptom that causes concern is intensely personal. From then on, if the symptom persists and the need is felt to seek advice or help, the person becomes the central point of an ever-widening circle which spreads out to involve more and more people. The person and confidant(s) reflect on the situation, and often refer to previous experiences which are perceived to be relevant. Advice and support are offered. Coping strategies are employed by the person in an attempt to control the symptoms and the individual's own reactions to their presence and perceived significance. All the time, as the circle widens, more and more information is received and meaning is attached to what is occurring. Eventually, after hours, days or months, medical personnel – the general practitioner, perhaps a physician, and finally the surgeon – enter the circle and, from then

on, have a major influence on events. Now there is an official interpretation of the problem. Eventually, the decision to operate is
made by a surgeon and agreed to by the patient.

Three concepts which will have a major influence on the work
of both patient and nurse have been developed from the field data:
Surfacing the Problem, Preparing for Intervention, and Interpreting the Experience.

Surfacing the Problem[3]

Unusual bleeding, a lump, a discharge, pain, indigestion, fatigue,
loss of weight – all are possible triggers to perception of a problem.
At this point the person is immediately involved in a process of
decision-making which concerns how to respond to the occurrence.
The outcome of this self-diagnostic process may be any of the
following decisions:

- No problem exists
- A problem may exist but it will not be acknowledged and no
  action will be taken
- A problem exists but requires no action
- A problem exists and vigilance is required to monitor it
- A problem exists and actions are available to resolve the problem
  within the person's own resources
- A problem exists and external consultation is necessary.

Decisions are influenced by the way in which the problem
presents and the significance attached to specific symptoms. Certain
phenomena produce an impact because they are are perceived as
life-threatening. Unusual bleeding, a lump or an unusual discharge
which appears suddenly is likely to cause alarm and initiate more
immediate action.

> The trouble is the blood . . . . I can't see anything but the blood.
> The first time it happened it really frightened me.

> About three weeks ago I noticed a lump here at the top of my leg
> . . . . and I rang the hospital . . .

> I woke up in the morning and found the discharge and panicked.

By contrast, symptoms such as indigestion, leg pain and those
associated with the presence of a hernia may be tolerated for
months, even years, before relief is finally sought through the
general practitioner.

> Nearly three years I have that. But it wasn't so bad last year. This year it started getting more heavy . . . . When I eat it sort of repeats and everything.

> Well, my legs started to play up and I'd walk about a hundred yards and they would start to ache, and I put up with that for about 18 months, and I thought I'd better go to the doctor and see if there is something wrong.

Indeed, it may even be that the doctor's decision for further action follows consultation on another unrelated matter.

> That's what I started off with – a leaky tap! And they knew the hernia was there, and they said, 'Oh well, we'd better get that fixed' . . . . I've known it's been there but it hasn't bothered me.

Because of nursing's focus on a person's moment-by-moment experience with the symptom(s) and the medical treatment regime, the pattern by which a problem surfaces is significant. There are four possible patterns associated with a problem surfacing: Evolution, Crisis On Evolution, Anticipated Crisis on Evolution, and Crisis.[4]

Each pattern has its own significance for the nursing care of a person throughout the subsequent hospitalisation and medical intervention.

Evolution: Nine of the 21 patients in this study presented a pattern of evolution which is characterised by the gradual development of a problem to the stage where non-urgent surgical intervention is recommended. While there may have been some initial apprehension about the meaning of the symptoms, fear of dire consequences has been alleviated following medical consultation. Despite this lack of a life-or-death crisis, the problem affects the world of the person into which it is intruding.

The evolutionary pattern involves:

- Duration of months or years
- Not presently associated with life threat
- Use of personal strategies to adjust to the presence of the problem, with variable success
- Alliance with the doctor for conservative management of the problem, often associated with periods of remission
- Referral to a surgeon as the problem persists
- Period of waiting for surgery.

There may be considerable diversity within the evolutionary pattern. Excerpts from the initial interviews of three of the nine patients who manifested this pattern are presented to illustrate this variability. The evolutionary process is apparent in both the history of the problem itself and each patient's adaptation to its continued presence.

A person with a five-year history of glaucoma:

> I don't think the illness in my eyes has made much difference to my lifestyle at all . . . . As long as I could put the drops in night and morning there didn't seem to be any problems . . . . According to Dr [ ] the pressure's increasing and he advised me to have the operation.

A person with a six-month history of rectal fissure:

> Yes, that's what it was − blood. I thought, 'Oh my God, I've got haemorrhoids!' Doctor said no, I had a fissure and he put me on suppositories and ointment. That worked for a while and he thought I was healing up and I had a relapse for a while. I was getting more and more uncomfortable and then he decided to refer me to a surgeon.

A person with a history from childhood of urinary tract infections:

> I just get bad kidney infections − you know − I can hardly walk and things like that. It's so common I just know when it's coming and when it's gone − you know. I used to go to the doctor all the time at home and he would just say, 'Oh yeah − problem child!' and feed me some more rubbish − antibiotics and stuff . . . . So that's why I thought I'd just come and get some more pills and that would be that. [Laughs] I didn't know that he was going to be on the ball!

When a person enters hospital and tells a story of their experience which seems to fit the dimensions of the evolutionary pattern, the nurse can recognise that this person has developed a degree of expertise in symptomatology. The person has lived with the progress of the condition, is probably aware of alternative treatment methods and may have been involved with one or more of these in alliance with the family doctor, has learned ways of adapting life style to cope with the effects of the symptoms and the demands of their conservative management, and is looking forward to the relief from symptoms which is anticipated after surgery.

Crisis On Evolution: Six of the 21 patients revealed a pattern of crisis following a period of evolution. Possibly over many years, the problem had surfaced according to the pattern of evolution. However, a critical turning point in the disease process has caused a change in the pattern which now manifests itself as:

- A recent change in a condition of long duration
- Presence of a life threat
- Personal coping strategies have become of increasingly limited effectiveness
- Previous alliance with the doctor for the conservative management of the problem
- Urgency attached to referral to the surgeon
- Urgency attached to admission for surgery.

Each of the six crises encountered in this study was unique and yet was consistent with the nature of the health problem. The crisis could originate as a dramatic development in the problem itself, such as the haemorrhaging associated with the development of oesophageal varices arising from chronic liver disease. Alternatively, a crisis may be precipitated by a traumatic event which influences that person's perspective on, and the status of, an evolving problem. Examples of this are the way in which grieving and subsequent loneliness may aggravate a chronic gastric ulcer, or the onset of a crisis when a patient with evolving cataracts which are complicating poor eyesight needs to learn self-dialysis for chronic renal disease.

In the following selections from interviews with two of the six people who demonstrated this pattern, it is possible to grasp the dramatic nature of the crisis and its impact on the person.

A person with oesophageal varices after a 15-year history of pain and indigestion since removal of her gallbladder:

> I get terrible gastro. Real pain towards the liver. This is where it all started. Always tender . . . . I take Aludrox most of the time now . . . . You do get the odd day when you could paint the moon but it will only last that one day and then you feel discomfort . . . . That pain has been there ever since the gallstones. I have never been one hundred percent since then – whatever happened then . . . . It's the pressure that built up evidently that perforated the thing and caused the haemorrhage . . . . I didn't expect it. I was having dinner . . . . I said, 'I don't feel like dinner' so I stopped eating and I said to my family, 'I'll go and lie down. I don't feel well.' I thought it was the flu. I think it was 7 o'clock that night I said, 'I think I'm going to be sick.' And I was absolutely amazed. I had had about three drinks of grape juice and I suppose that must have made the amount look

more. We rang the ambulance. It was a whole bowl full . . . . Came top and bottom . . . . I got an urge to pass and it was all black there. The other part was red . . . . The ambulance man took my blood pressure and he said it was absolutely high. They just crept along the road. He was afraid to go over a bump, he said, in case I exploded . . . . After three or four days, he [the physician] went down the throat again and that is when he decided he wanted Mr [the surgeon] to have a look at me. This thing has changed everything. I just don't know when it's going to happen.

This experience, consistent with the nature of the medical problem, illustrates the way in which a life-threatening crisis can affect a situation which has been evolving over many years. The patient's recognition of danger is evident in her words: 'Time is running out really, isn't it!'

A person who had had a gastric ulcer for 15 years and had been recently widowed:

I live on my own now. My wife died this year. I'm a lousy cook, I'll say that. [Laughs] This has probably not helped me over the last few months. Possibly I've aggravated my ulcer in the process but, anyway, I'll make out . . . . It's been a good 15 years since I was first diagnosed that I had an ulcer. That's when it started playing up . . . . She died on [date] and I suppose it was nerves. I don't know what aggravated it. I started losing weight. I think I look after myself alright. I can't cook but I found that you have to learn to do these things. Everything started up again as far as my problem was concerned and it just wouldn't settle down. I lost a lot of weight – about two stone . . . . I was sick so much, I think . . . . when I went to bed I would get a buildup of acidity and I finished up vomiting every night.

This man associated the critical deterioration in his physical condition with the recent death of his wife. An exacerbation of symptoms associated with his chronic gastric ulcer had ensued which, accompanied by persistent vomiting and marked loss of weight, led to real concern for his health.

As with the evolutionary pattern, the person with this pattern of crisis has been living with the condition, often for a period of years. The impact of the chronic condition on the person's life may have meant that considerable adjustment in many aspects of daily living has been required. A variety of treatment regimes may have been attempted which would require the person's concentrated effort in an alliance with the doctor. Expertise in the symptomatology and progress of the condition is apparent. New dimensions of urgency and a feeling of threat now influence the behaviour of the patient as surgery approaches.

Anticipated Crisis on Evolution: Examination of the patients' stories revealed a particular pattern of evolution in which the nature of the gradual disease process was one which they knew could, indeed probably would, eventually culminate in a fearful event such as death, a severe heart attack or a debilitating stroke. This pattern is usually associated with pathological changes in the walls of the arteries. In each of the two patients exhibiting this pattern, the blood vessels supplying the brain were becoming increasingly narrowed and damaged by arteriosclerosis with the probability that this would eventually lead to a stroke. Other major vessels may be involved, particularly the coronary arteries.

Advances in medical science now make it possible to diagnose and to treat such progressive conditions before the threatened event occurs. Thus, people with this problem are able to visualise a possible future of death or debilitation if the condition is untreated. They have to decide whether or not to accept the major surgery which could prevent a future crisis.

In practice, while a degree of urgency is attached to the need for this surgery, the actual waiting time for admission to hospital may be considerably longer due to the lack of treatment resources available and the number of people waiting for the same preemptive surgery. This may be perceived as paradoxical, even conflicting. While the waiting continues, the threat persists. This persisting threat means that death or serious disability could occur at any time.

This pattern presents as:

- Either a life-threatening event such as a heart attack or minimal awareness of symptoms but evidence of generalised arterial disease
- Possibility of life threat or disability without medical intervention
- Personal coping strategies fully utilised to control uncertainty and apprehension
- Degree of urgency attached to referral to surgeon
- Urgency attached to need for surgery followed by a period of waiting for weeks to months for admission.

Extracts from the initial interview with one of the two people who exhibited this pattern is presented to illustrate the characteristic pattern.

A person with an 18-month history of pain in his legs during exercise:

> Well, my legs started to play up and I'd walk about a hundred yards and they would start to ache, and I put up with that for about 18 months and I thought I'd better go to the doctor to see if there is something wrong. I'd walk a hundred yards and have to stop . . . then it would go away. Anyway it wound up that I have circulation problems . . . . He [the general practitioner] sent me to [the surgeon] and they checked me, done me all over and advised me to have a test, which I did and it proved positive that I should have an operation. So here I am!

This man later confirmed that he had agreed to the surgery because of his fear of the threat posed by this condition.

> . . . [the surgeon] says, 'The blood goes up one side and down the other down there,' he says, 'and they are closing up, and,' he said, 'they will get to a stage where you will have a stroke.' So that convinced me. I says, 'Well right – whatever, whenever.' That's about the operation . . . . If I was to have a stroke it's going to be curtains . . . . I have seen a few people with them – not me!

While the disease processes of the two patients who manifested this pattern were similar, their personal circumstances, of real significance to nursing, were very different. For example, one man had experienced a recent family tragedy with continuing problems, while the other had previously experienced a heart attack, had been required to journey from a nearby town for the surgery and, because his children lived overseas and his wife could not drive, would have no family visiting during his hospitalisation. However, the probable future crisis and the strong desire to prevent it were almost identical.

When such patients are admitted to hospital for planned surgery they will be anticipating the removal of a threat. The consequences of the threat becoming a reality are known through the experiences of others – perhaps sudden death, or a stroke, or a massive heart attack. All are to be feared and prevented if at all possible. The decision to accept surgical intervention involves an intellectual decision as well as an emotional response. Thus, the person has decided that, although there may be no current problems, the threat is serious enough to warrant acceptance of the doctor's recommendation for major surgery.

Crisis: Four of the 21 patients in this study demonstrated a pattern of crisis. All were women. The crises involved the sudden presentation of a possible malignancy. Perception of the future when cancer is a possibility includes visions of pain and suffering before inevitable death. Future plans are in turmoil. Uncertainty becomes the prevalent feeling.

This crisis pattern presents as:

- Possible or proven malignancy which has become apparent only recently
- Awareness of a proven or potential life threat
- Personal coping strategies fully utilised to control apprehension over outcome of surgery
- Urgency attached to referral to the surgeon
- Urgency attached to admission for surgery.

A crisis pattern arises from the way the presenting problem affects the daily life of the person. All of a sudden there is a threat which might necessitate a rethinking of present and future plans. While there may be an existing health problem, the crisis-inducing problem is usually unrelated and may arise without warning. At the time of admission the future is uncertain. Hope is held that the surgery will remove the threat but it is also realised, with some apprehension, that surgery may not be successful.

Despite the similarity of the actual problem – cancer – and the common acknowledgement of a sense of panic or shock, the individual circumstances of each person cause variations in the experience. This is well illustrated in the following excerpts from interviews with two of the four women concerned.

A person with a discharge from the nipple:

> I woke up in the morning and found the discharge and panicked – about a month ago. Rang up my doctor and Nurse said he was busy and couldn't take me till the next day unless it was urgent. So I said I don't know whether it's urgent or not but I have a discharge from the nipple and I'm panicking. So she said, 'Come at 12 o'clock' . . . . By 3.30 I was being interviewed in the hospital here . . . . He passed me on that quickly. Both doctors at the time said there was only a very small percentage of people that did have cancer, who came and thought it was a possibility . . . . Last Thursday, the day of the

operation biopsy, not the needle one, a few hours beforehand . . . they put a needle into where the spot showed in the x-ray . . . and they left it there until they operated later in the day and took the lump out and had it examined and it was found to be malignant. So that's the stage I'm at now . . . . Everyone says I'm marvellous but I just can't believe I've got anything wrong with me because – I mean I know I have – but it hasn't sunk in. Because I feel so well. I'm still hungry – putting on a bit of weight if I'm not careful – and panic in between times of course.

This elderly woman had been involved in repeated personal crises over recent months. In addition to the crisis induced by the presence of malignancy, admission to hospital created home management problems and did not reduce concern about her family situation. During the conversation, she raised the issue of a possible link between her personal stress and the onset of the malignancy when she stated, 'I would like to have asked if worry brings on cancer in any way.'

A person with a history of Hodgkin's disease 20 years before and a melanoma two years previously:

Then two years ago I had that melanoma which was a bit of a shock because I thought everything was going so well. About three weeks ago I noticed a bit of a lump here at the top of my leg in the groin and I rang the hospital and I came to go to [the surgeon]. That was last Tuesday and the doctor there said he would have to put me into hospital this week and have it removed. That was another bit of a shock. I just felt I was getting over this foot . . . . It was just the shock of coming in when you think everything is going so well.

In this example, the crisis represents the first indication that the original cancer has spread from the foot. Despite her history, the crisis still came unexpectedly after a period of apparent recovery. The crisis is perhaps even more important in this situation because it comes after a lot of hard work and hope on the part of this woman – following orders, adapting lifestyle, thinking through the issue of having cancer, appearing to have conquered it, beginning to look to the future and suddenly having to rethink everything as a new threat appears. Also, there is evidence of some continuing concern about the health of her husband and about his ability to cope in her absence. Her concern for her own frail mother, who was staying with her at the time of discovering the lump, added another complication.

All of the people showing the crisis pattern in this study

became aware of a visible lump or discharge. This is not always the first sign. Interviews with other people suggest that many experience an initial pattern of non-specific "unwellness" or another sign or symptom which could occur with a number of conditions. For example, two patients interviewed later had experienced a feeling of lethargy and general ill health with the later sign of mild jaundice for months preceding admission. One other had had constipation for two years despite many attempted remedies, while another had abdominal discomfort with a feeling of being bloated. As the picture persisted and intensified, further medical examinations eventually raised the spectre of malignancy, and thus crisis.

The crisis pattern by which a problem surfaces brings a person into nursing care at a time of panic. A sense of urgency and crisis has been reinforced by the words and actions of the medical staff. The outcome, if the problem is left untreated, is feared. Surgery is seen as essential and welcomed in order to avoid the threat of pain, suffering and death, even though the surgery itself may be life-threatening and/or could alter the person's body image. Thus, hope comes in the form of an opportunity to choose radical medical intervention.

These four patterns refer to more than the actual development of a physiological anomaly. They encompass the integration of the problem into the daily life of the person, and include the actions and reactions of the person as the situation unfolds. The person who enters the Nursing Partnership as part of the process of resolving the problem brings this experience along.

Preparing for Intervention

When a surgeon recommends surgery, and the person agrees to this action, a period of planning ensues. Plans are made in relation to home, family, job and other responsibilities; night clothes are checked and new ones may be purchased. There is a general preparation for a temporary withdrawal from the usual pattern of daily living.

In addition, each person gets ready to become a patient and undergo surgery. This aspect of the preparation will be influenced by the way in which the problem has surfaced. In particular, the presence of a perceived threat to life affects the way the upcoming experience is approached. Analysis of the initial interviews revealed that, during this period, people strive to achieve a state of acquiescence, associated with equanimity and order within themselves and their own world.

Acquiescence, in this context, is defined as 'agreement without protest' to a course of action which involves personal suffering in order to achieve a goal perceived to be beneficial (Collins, 1979). It includes the belief that the right decision has been made, as well as the development of confidence in the surgeon responsible. During the initial interviews it became apparent that there was also a widespread distinctive quality of dignity, composure, serenity and calmness – that is, equanimity – which people seemed to perceive as the appropriate approach to hospitalisation and surgery. Interviews at the time of admission revealed that most people had been able to attain this state, even when in a crisis pattern.

The following examples show that some people accept surgery in the anticipation of relief from troublesome symptoms.

> . . . I just finished up vomiting every night . . . . They just have to do something about it the way it was going. Well, they did, too, because I would have finished up a physical wreck probably . . . . Fortunately, I hope or have been assured that they can make a new man of me!

> It appears there's a bit of tissue there that's causing the problem and the only way to get over it is to chop it out . . . . Whatever will be will be. If it's got to be done, let's get the darned thing over and done with.

Each person in the study seemed to be assured that the surgery was necessary and all but one appeared to be composed in preparation for the surgical experience. The woman who had failed to attain this goal before admission had an unusual prelude period which was exacerbated by the need to change her surgeon due to his illness. Her acknowledged anxiety about the possibility of cancer was heightened by the delays in medical appointments caused by the change in surgeon. Finally, after pressure from her, and because of a cancellation, she was admitted at relatively short notice. According to her own account, this scenario left her in an unsettled state at the time of admission.

> I felt that no one was looking after me and I was extremely anxious . . . . I had seen [the surgeon] for a couple of minutes and unfortunately he became ill and no one has seen me except this registrar and I just felt he was not up to it. I had no faith in him at all . . . . he's a couple of years older than me . . . . When I came in here this morning I just freaked out.

Nursing action was required to give specific assistance to this person.

The research data also revealed that composure was associated with denial of the presence of worry or anxiety about the upcoming surgery by the majority of patients.

> I certainly have the greatest respect and no fears about [the surgeon].

> It doesn't really worry me. I thought, 'Oh well, you know what you're doing.'

> This time I'm not worrying – no. In fact, I might even be looking forward to it.

Some people may experience a specific fear or concern associated with the problem itself, as distinct from the surgery. In the following two examples, one man shared his feeling of unease that the death of another person was making his surgery possible, and an elderly woman spoke of her fears about cancer.

> I think one of the other things about this particular operation which I find – peculiar – it gives me a funny feeling – is that they term it – 'You've got to wait for suitable material!' – which means you've got to wait for someone else to be killed off. Okay – what will be will be. If they're going to die, they're going to die. But I still find it very hard to accept or – I suppose I accept it – but I find it hard to take the fact that, for my benefit, the whole thing relies on something unfortunate happening to someone else. It's not a pleasant feeling . . . . It's started now . . . . I think probably a mixture of a bit of nausea, I suppose, and gratitude amongst it.

> 'Got to get rid of it,' [the surgeon] told me. I was flabbergasted. I'm a bit nervous coming back here today. Stomach's a bit wiggly-wobbly.

For some the concern arose from their personal circumstances.

> When I found out I was sick my biggest alarm was how was [ ] going to get on without me . . . . So I'm worried from that point of view.

Rather than presenting overt anxiety, almost all subjects demonstrated humour during the initial interview when recounting their story. Humour may be very informative to the listening nurse as it reveals the patient's past and present feelings and reactions. Three excerpts are given to illustrate this point.

I live on my own now. My wife died this year. I'm a lousy cook, I'll say that!

He showed me the x-rays and said, 'Oh yeah, you'll have to come into hospital,' and I thought, 'Oh yeah, me and my big mouth!'

The surgeon said, 'You don't have to worry very much. They're doing this operation on the streets of Bombay with a bamboo stick so it can't be that bad. Mind you, it hurts a bit!' So that reassured me, so long as it's not done by those means in this hospital!

The prevalence of composure with good humour suggests that persons who are about to undergo surgery perceive a social expectation that they present themselves in this way.

Although this image of a desirable state arose from the data, the nature of the research gives little explanation of the reason. It seemed to be important to people that others perceive them as being in control of themselves. Even if there is uncertainty or fear underneath, the outward appearance of calm contributes to the maintenance of self-esteem within the person. If uncertainty and/or lack of equanimity remains at the time of admission, urgency is attached to overcoming this immediately after entry into the Nursing Partnership. This urgency arises from the patient's need to settle issues which are causing concern so that maximum resources can be focused on the surgery itself.

Interpreting the Experience

As new experiences unfold people attempt to attach meaning to every event and incorporate it, together with their reactions, into the integrated story of their life. Thus, there is a constant process of analysis and synthesis.

By the time patients enter hospital, they have put this personalised interpretation of their experience in a form which can be shared with others. From the multitude of experiences, reactions and feelings which contribute to the story a selection has been made of what are considered to be the critical issues. This is then recounted in turn to family or friends, the general practitioner, the surgeon, perhaps other medical staff and the nurse. Each time the story is told the person receives comments and reactions which will be interpreted and may be included in subsequent versions of the story. Thus, the story continues to change and develop, perhaps becoming more complex, perhaps containing less omissions, as more information is received.

In this study it quickly became obvious that there was considerable variation in the completeness of patients' accounts of their experience and in the desire of each person to fill in the gaps even when these were recognised. Omissions in the story were often associated with the intended action by the surgeon to remedy the problem. This is demonstrated in the following exchange between the researcher and one person.

And do you understand what you have come in for – what do you think you have come in for?

I don't really know.

When you were talking it over with [the surgeon], did he explain it to you?

Oh he just showed me the x-ray and he says he's going to . . . I think something's blocked and he's going to unblock it.

Mm.

So that's why I thought it was only going to take a couple of days and I'd be home again.

Did you think they would go in from below or . . .?

Well, no. I hoped from down here [points to mouth] but I really thought from below. I thought that might happen. I really didn't know.

And you didn't want to ask?

No. I just thought, 'Oh well, when I come here they'll tell me, I guess.' 'Cause it's horrible people pestering you all the time. 'Cause, you know, there's people at work like that – What are you doing? What are you doing? – you know. It gets me riled. So I thought, 'Just wait, he'll tell me.'

So you're quite happy with that?

Yeah. I don't care. I didn't even know how many days I'd be in for. I thought two.

That's the sort of thing you should ask if you want to know the answer.

Yeah.

When the doctors come round they will probably ask you how much you know – and then its up to you.

Yeah. It doesn't really worry me. I thought, 'Oh well, you know what you're doing.'

This example illustrates some people's reticence to actively seek information even when key questions remain unanswered and the story is incomplete. Such an open acknowledgement of ignorance was made by eight subjects in this study group during the first interview, and most of these seemed to be willing to accept that their lack of knowledge was to be expected. Indeed, the points of ignorance and the belief that this was to be expected were incorporated into the story. Knowledge and expertise are attributed to the medical staff. The following exchange illustrates this point.

> Well, they're going to do my neck first. I don't know what they do. And after a week or two they do the leg.
>
> Why do you have to have an operation on your neck?
>
> I wouldn't have a clue. It's all to do with the circulation.
>
> So you've come into hospital expecting that you are going to have one operation on your neck and then, a little bit later, an operation on your leg. Is that right?
>
> As far as I understand. They just give you the bare facts, I think. They don't go into detail.
>
> Would you like them to go into detail or are you happy with that?
>
> It's all the same to me.

One elderly woman with a life-threatening condition showed a marked variation from this pattern by repeatedly expressing a wish to know more about her situation. Even when sharing this with the researcher, this woman was always extremely composed, speaking very quietly and deliberately without overt anxiety.

> I don't know much about it. They don't tell you a lot. I often think they should tell you more.
>
> You don't feel you can ask?
>
> Well, I have asked and I don't seem to get anywhere. They sort of shove you off. They do really! All they say is we must get you well and all the rest of it.

Later:

> I know very little about it even though I have had the experience, but I wish they would tell you more. [The physician] put me before a panel of doctors in Ward [   ] and they were asking me about the gallbladder operation. I couldn't tell them much about it because [the previous surgeon] never explained much to me. I was quite

> content to let things lie. He said, 'She has a very chronic liver complaint.' That's the first time I ever heard it was bad. I wish they would tell you that little bit more.

Paradoxically, this patient seemed sincere when she spoke of her high regard for the medical staff, particularly the physician with overall management of her disease, in spite of comments regarding her lack of knowledge.

> He has been absolutely wonderful to me. So interested. And he has done everything he could for me. As he said, 'We have got to get you well – well, as well as we can.'

There was considerable variation in the terminology used by people to recount their stories. Some used medical terminology, others translated the story into language that was personally meaningful. No pattern was found in the unstructured interviews in this study to account for the variation among the subjects.

There was some evidence of wisdom about diseases, tests, the hospital and staff that arose from continuing association with the health professions by those who had a chronic disease and by those who had experienced previous surgical intervention for the same problem. However, there was no consistency among this group on the nature of the terminology used. Short excerpts from the stories of three people who had had considerable contact with health professionals in recent years are presented to demonstrate the variation in language.

A person with a breast lump:

> . . . they operated later in the day and took the lump out and had it examined and it was found to be malignant.

A person in hospital for a second corneal graft and a history of eye problems since childhood:

> He [a doctor consulted while overseas] said there was a cut on the cornea. I asked him if it was an old one or a new one. He couldn't tell. I suspect it was an old one because it cleared up . . . . It appears there's a bit of bad tissue there that's causing the problem and the only way to get over it is to chop it out.

A person with an eight-year history of renal failure requiring home dialysis:

> [The surgeon] said those three things should be cured by this parathyroidectomy . . . . I take a lot of pills to lower the calcium

level – Titralac, Cemetidine and others to try and lower it. They must have done because the levels today are good. I tried to explain to the doctor that electrolyte levels taken after dialysis are never correct. She said they were good. I said you should take them tomorrow. That's the day when they settle down again and you'll see what they really are.

Analysis of the initial interviews in this study indicates that the way in which people recount the story of their experience and expectations is very important. The demeanour, the language used, the way in which potential life threats or crises are discussed, the topics chosen for inclusion or given emphasis, the spontaneous expressions of 'not knowing' and reactions to this – all these give the nurse invaluable insight into the world of the person as perceived at the time of admission to hospital and entry into the Nursing Partnership.

Events which precede a person's entry into hospital and into the Nursing Partnership proper have been portrayed as the Beginning. Each person entering the state of 'being nursed' has a Beginning experience which is shared with others in its component processes, but which is unique as a synthesised whole.

[1] Footnotes will be used to explain the origin of the terminology used in each concept.

[2] The term 'beginning' was coined to reflect the fact that the Nursing Partnership actually has its origins in the prelude period before admission. Its form is consistent with the gerundial terminology used throughout the framework to reflect ongoing process.

[3] The term 'surfacing', with its dictionary meaning of 'emerging' or 'becoming apparent', reflects the constant references by patients to their complex experiences of living with the problem prior to admission (Collins, 1979).

[4] The terms 'evolution' and 'crisis' reflect both the development of the problem through time and its present impact on the life of the person. Evolution is defined as 'a gradual development' which requires a degree of adaptation and adjustment but is not life-threatening. By contrast, crisis is used to denote 'a sudden change for the worse' – a decisive event which presents a major threat to the person's outlook on, and expectation of, life (Collins, 1979). This crisis is 'situational', as it occurs 'as a result of some unanticipated traumatic event that is usually beyond one's control' (Hoff, 1978, p 12).

[5] This term describes the preparatory behaviour patients revealed in interviews.

[6] This term denotes analysing and information-sharing behaviour patients revealed in interviews.

4   ENTERING THE NURSING
PARTNERSHIP – SETTLING IN

By reporting to the Admission Office, completing and signing the admission documentation, a person presenting for elective surgery becomes an in-patient of the hospital. Thereafter, instructions are given on how to proceed to the assigned surgical ward. Entry into the ward, the domain of the nursing staff, symbolises entry into the Nursing Partnership. A period of transition now begins for the patient from a state of 'not being nursed' to a state of 'being nursed'.

People vary in their degree of unfamiliarity with being a patient in hospital, with the experience of surgery, and with receiving nursing. For example, five people in this study had had the same or a related operation in the same ward within the last two years. In contrast, for three this was the first admission to hospital for any reason. Between these two extremes lay the experiences of 13 others, some of whom were familiar with other wards in the hospital as a result of their admission in recent years for other or related health conditions. Whatever the individual's previous experience, each person faces the task of adjusting to the new situation.

From the moment of the first encounter with nursing staff, patients begin the process of negotiating their own passage with the specialised assistance of the nurse. This negotiating work is discussed later. There is also a separate but concurrent process of initiation into the Nursing Partnership: Settling In.[1]

There are two participants in the process of Settling In – the patient and the nurse. The work of the patient is to make the transition to becoming a patient – in relation to the hospital, the medical staff, other health professionals and the nursing staff. The work of the nurse is to facilitate this process. In the remainder of this chapter the work of patient and nurse during Settling In will be presented with illustrations selected from the data to support each concept.

Settling In: The Work of the Patient

Families, homes, social worlds and the usual pattern of daily living are left behind when people enter hospital. The Nursing Partnership assists the individual to become a patient, to adapt to the new setting and status, and to prepare for the upcoming experience of surgery.

From the field data three separate but interrelated areas of patient work have been identified: Becoming a Patient, Suspending Social Roles, and Revealing Self. Each one will be discussed with supportive excerpts which are primarily drawn from patient interviews.

Becoming a Patient[2]

While being called 'patient' from the outset, people 'become' patients through a complex pattern of discovery and learning as well as a preparedness to open themselves to the unknown. No matter how often a person has been a patient in the past, even in the same ward, there is always something new in each experience – new problems, new personal and family circumstances, new faces, new procedures, new decor, and so on.

From their first contact with the patient, nursing staff members are easing their way into the role and its required work by selecting, translating and sharing necessary information with the patient. Helpful information includes the physical layout of the ward, the names of key personnel, how to order meals, and how to contact the nursing staff.

> I've only shown him around and given him directions and spoken to him . . .

Some patients spoke of the value their previous experiences of being a patient were at this time. Such people already possessed some of the information required to settle into the ward and into the Nursing Partnership.

> I'm finding it much easier. I know what's sort of going to happen . . . . I think knowing what the routine was is quite helpful.

However, a previous experience may actually impede a patient's Settling In. For example, one patient had had the same operation in another hospital several years before and found his admission experience very confusing.

> When I had the other graft done they were so careful about infection and everything and when I come in here there seems to be a complete change of philosophy . . . . I'm assuming I'll stay here, in this bed, this cubicle – I'm assuming at this point – which I find quite strange after the other two experiences. But everyone to his job. I'm no expert. If it's safe and what they did in the old days, it wasn't necessary, then I leave it to their judgement . . . . I still find it hard to understand but I accept it.

In the formal preoperative teaching session on the day of admission, this man set out to uncover any further conflict by not disclosing the knowledge he already possessed and permitting the nurse to 'teach' him again.

> I asked some questions that I knew the answers to, but I was interested to see what their answers would be.

Confusion could also be induced by inconsistent information from hospital personnel. One patient later reported she had been given three different predictions on the duration of her stay in hospital – two, seven and 15 days. Another patient was given information by nursing staff which inferred she would be having an abdominal wound, but later that day the registrar informed her that this would not be the case.

> But everyone's been telling me today, 'You're being cut', then this other guy comes along and says, 'You're not being cut'. They're going to go up through my bladder. So I don't know what it is now . . . . Oh, it doesn't really matter. It'll be in the morning anyway.

A significant part of becoming a patient is accepting the reality that a reliance on the expertise of others will be necessary in order to achieve the goal which caused the entry to hospital. Indeed, there is an active willingness to follow rules and undergo unpleasant, uncomfortable and/or undignified procedures in order to maximise the chances of a successful outcome. One patient assured the researcher of his cooperation with whatever was required.

> I'll stick to the rules.

However, throughout the study it became clear that, although this apparent submission was common, it was neither passive nor complete. In the following example, from an interview on the evening of admission, the patient was reflecting on his sense of powerlessness and his feeling that 'they' had taken over. Paradoxically, at the same time he was able to recount an experience in which he did exert control, when given the opportunity.

> There is nothing I can do. It's in their hands so you just have to carry on with what they do and go along . . . . It's a fact. It's going to happen regardless . . . . You have got to accept it . . . . They asked me if I wanted one [sleeping pill] but I don't believe in them . . . . If the body needs sleep, it will have sleep . . . . I'll wait until it comes on to me and then I'll go off. No, I don't want any sleeping pills or anything like that.

Encounters with medical and nursing students may occur in the Settling In period. Soon after admission, any patient might be asked to give assistance to basic and graduate students as they gain experience or as they prepare for examinations. Patients gave the impression that they were willing to cooperate with learning activities associated with a teaching hospital, even when 'learning' was the only purpose for a procedure. However, despite their assent to such intrusions, the patients demonstrated that they were evaluating the behaviour of the learner.

> I feel a bit like a guinea pig . . . . Two lots have looked into the eye – at the eye. The before and after stages they wanted to have a look at . . . .

> Later: I was rather amused. They put in the Chloramphenicol and said, 'Don't put your fingers in your eye. If you get tears, wipe it with a tissue.' That goes in every three hours, and in the meantime you get about four or five doctors prodding and touching.

> . . . Dr [   ] came along and wanted to examine me and I said yes. He's taking an exam tomorrow . . . . Yes, he seemed very nervous. He did a full three-quarters of an hour investigation without me telling him what the trouble was, you know. He diagnosed it all. That was a bit wearying, I suppose. And then the Pakistani doctor came and took me away for a quarter of an hour and went through the same procedure! . . . .

> Later: The trouble is, quite frankly, the doctors come and interrupt the nurses in their work. The charge nurse [actually staff nurse] was sitting down to give me a preoperative counselling and this guy comes along and says, 'Do you mind?' – so he wheels me away and she's left like a shag on a rock and has to come back and do it this evening. It's the old coordination. I don't think doctors should have unrestricted access to patients at all hours when it suits them!

Patients are able to recognise expertise as well as its absence. The former engenders confidence, the latter unease. In the following example the patient knew the surgeon was away and was reassured only after a conversation with another surgeon who told her he would be present at her surgery.

> In fact, I didn't even know he was going to do it. I thought Dr [   ] was involved. In the back of my mind I thought he was a bit young – a bit inexperienced, perhaps – seeing [the surgeon] was away and he was just his helper . . . . So I was, in some ways, quite relieved when [the surgeon] came along.

Patients' relationships with experts and their maintenance of equanimity will be developed further in Chapter 5.

Becoming a patient involves: selective submission which is associated with an ability to distinguish experts from learners; retention of a degree of assertiveness; an acceptance of personal responsibility to contribute to the outcome; and a willingness to cooperate from the moment of admission. During this time patients attempt to understand what is expected of them as they prepare to undergo the ordeal of surgery.

Suspending Social Roles[3]

Each person who becomes a patient has already learned to present a 'face' to the world that allows survival in the individual's social world and physical setting. At no time is the 'real' self totally exposed. While socialising in the community, the individual learns the skills associated with daily living. These include strategies consistent with the prevailing pattern of beliefs and customs within that social group. At any time, a person occupies a number of social roles – such as those in relation to family, work, religion and recreation – and these roles make demands but also confirm that person's place in the world.

Admission to hospital, and the effects of treatment measures such as surgery, cause a person to change, at least temporarily, this daily pattern of living and interacting with the world, whatever the cultural background. Usual roles and responsibilities must be shed or modified when the role of hospital patient is assumed. Hospitalisation also requires the patient to relinquish a large degree of independence and privacy.

In this study, a marked sense of responsibility, associated with the need to be absent from social roles during the period of hospitalisation and rehabilitation, was evident during discussions with the patients at the time of admission. The following three examples reflect the prevailing sense of commitment by patients to ensure that their usual areas of responsibility are exercised by others in their absence.

> I'm what they call the floor warden there too . . . . I didn't have a deputy. I lost him because he went downstairs to another floor. I had to appoint another one yesterday – just in case . . . . Also, I had to show the civil defence . . .

> . . . of course, when I found out I was sick my biggest alarm was how was [the ill husband] going to get on without me. But we've got a daughter and she's holding the fort.

> I started to try and organise things and complete things so, if I did disappear in a hurry, it wouldn't cause too much disruption . . . . So you've got to make it so that whoever does the thing [work] on your behalf is as well equipped as they possibly can be.

Prior to hospitalisation there is often a time of increased activity in order to hand over responsibility to others. It is possible that the person may be tired from this effort on arrival to the hospital. An example of this is the following exchange with one person several hours after admission.

> I was sleeping before.

> Did you just feel tired and doze off?

> Just felt tired and dozed off.

> Had you been doing extra work at work to get ready to come or something?

> No, not so much at work but I've been doing stuff at home.

> I see, you mean like mowing the lawns . . .

> Concreting!

> Oh my goodness.

> Concreting the garage floor – digging it all out and I was putting a concrete floor down before I came in so the car could come in off the road while I'm away.

The full or partial suspension of the person's usual social roles and the assumption of the patient role is common to all patients, but its details – the constellation of roles, the concerns about their maintenance during the period of hospitalisation and recovery, the ability to withdraw from each role and the personal investment in the roles – are specific to each person.

Revealing Self[4]

During the time of Settling In, patients are faced with the need to shed the privacy that normally surrounds their person and personal affairs. Access to personal information about their bodies, as well as daily life and circumstances, are sought by the health professionals as a part of their work. In addition, hospital practices demand changes in behaviour which expose aspects of a person's living pattern which are normally reserved for home and family.

For example, nightwear is usually worn at home, at night. In hospital it is worn all the time. No patient expressed concern about this. Indeed, people enter hospital expecting to wear night clothes and most come prepared with enough nightwear to last during their time in hospital. This expectation is validated by the behaviour of nurses during the admission procedure, who tend to show the person to a bed, pull the screens and ask the person to change into night attire before any further action is taken.

> I came up here just as they were having a cup of tea . . . and after that I changed and put on my dressing gown and pyjamas and then they came in and checked off my clothes.

In everyday living, privacy of the person also involves restricting access by others to the sight and touch of the body and body discharges. The degree of restriction is socially and culturally determined although there is considerable individual variation. However, this restriction is relaxed when a person is in the care of a nurse. This willingness to shed privacy seems to arise from an acceptance of the legitimacy of the nurse's role in relation to the care of a person's body. No negative comment or disquiet was expressed by the people in this study concerning the nurses' actions in this regard. Indeed, patients seemed to tolerate this unmasking with equanimity right from admission so that procedures like weighing, often deliberately done in private at home, were willingly undertaken in public. Even usually concealed body discharges, such as urine, were handed over to nursing staff.

During Settling In, the patient often submits to intrusive activities related to the upcoming surgery. Some are performed by the doctor – rectal examination, vaginal examination, breast examination, for example. Others are performed by the nurse.

Nurse has just shaved me ready for the morning [pubic shave].

I had an enema last night only because she told me it would be a good idea.

Even the consequences of such procedures are regarded with composure, and occasionally humour. One elderly man had a twinkle in his eye as he described the unpleasant aftermath of an enema as being 'just like the old tune *Annie Laurie* – she played on!'

The initiation rites performed by nurses bring them into close contact with the patient. Normal patterns of self-care are probed with particular emphasis on identifying areas where special nursing assistance will be required. In the data were examples of patients: who found it difficult to move freely around the house and had developed coping strategies for that setting; who struggled to reach all body areas while in the shower; who had difficulty dressing because of imperfect functioning and/or painful joints; and who had difficulty reaching the toilet during the night. It was evident that such problems might have relevance for nursing even when the adaptive strategies used by the patient meant they were no longer perceived as problems under normal circumstances. For example, the researcher, as nurse, observed that one patient had no dentures, assumed they had been left at home and anticipated that this could be a problem in relation to hospital meals.

> You didn't tell me about them this morning. [Researcher had already telephoned son to ask him to bring in hearing aid]
>
> No. I didn't tell you about them at all. [Patient chuckles]
>
> Do you feel better not wearing them?
>
> Well, I'm not retching or vomiting. That's the trouble.
>
> You have pretty soft food – everything mashed up?
>
> Oh no, I can eat it as long as I chop it through a bit . . . . I'm quite happy without them.

Each person has some areas of personal privacy which may need to be revealed, partially or completely, in word or by sight, to the nurse during this hospital experience. Acceptance of this kind of exposure is associated with the required acquiescence. Nurses are accepted as being one group of people to whom it is safe to expose these areas of perceived vulnerability in order to receive assistance as required.

During discussion with the nurse, a patient may reveal much more personal information than the nurse seeks. Nurses, who minutes before were strangers, may gain a very intimate insight into the world of the patient. One man cried during the initial interview when talking about his daily life since his wife had died, and went on to speak of how he had coped.

> I thought I had got over that . . . . I have a bit of a garden and a bit of lawn to do, so by the time I do the house and make the meals and do the garden, that occupies the mornings and the bowls occupy the afternoon. The evenings are the only time I find a little bit quiet. Pull the blinds down and shut yourself off from the rest of the world.

Such information is precious to the person and its revelation reflects the immediate closeness which characterises the contact between nurses and patients within the Nursing Partnership – even though they are actually strangers.

Admission to hospital is also associated with an openness between patients, particularly in the area of health status and the upcoming surgery.

> . . . he's having the same operation . . . he had this eye done three years ago . . . he said it's totally different than last time.

> When I came home [from the outpatient clinic] I thought about it and discussed it at home and everyone one I talked to – which wasn't many because I didn't like to tell the world about my medical history. It's funny, when you get in here you forget all about that. You like to know what everyone else has got . . .

There is a camaraderie born of the shared experience that seems to begin immediately. Indeed, advice is offered by people who were complete strangers a short while before but are now considered allies and even friends.

> My fellow contemporary over there thought I should have one [sleeping pill].

Revealing self seems to be a key task for the patient while settling into the Nursing Partnership. This is a vulnerable transition as the patient exposes personal information about self and circumstances to strangers. Support for this process of unusual openness comes from fellow patients, family, and friends as well as the hospital staff. However, at all times the patient retains some control over the amount of revealing done. While no person lays bare their total being to anyone, patients accept that nurses have the right of access to highly personal information for the purpose of rendering nursing assistance.

Settling In: The Work of the Nurse

The nurse performs the rites that mark the patient's initiation into the Nursing Partnership. At this time the nurse seeks to add a nursing component to settling the patient into the hospital, the ward and the care of other personnel who will intermittently deal with the patient. Analysis of the field data revealed two separate but co-existing areas in which nursing is working during the Settling In period: Admitting, and Appraising.

Admitting[5]

Admitting comprises a routine of specific tasks which nurses perform on behalf of others. While these provide information for the patient during admission to a surgical ward, they are also a major source of information from the patient. From the nursing documentation and nurse interviews in this study, it became clear that the tasks involved in this area of nursing work can be divided into two groups: those which provide baseline data of primary value to the medical management of the patient, such as temperature, pulse, respiration, blood pressure, weight and urinalysis; and those performed on behalf of the institution, such as security of clothing, labelling of records and ordering of meals.

The Admitting ritual may be recorded in the nursing documentation as a partial or full checklist of tasks. Those remaining uncompleted at the end of the admitting nurse's period of duty may be specially noted to remind the next shift that they are still to be done. Entries in the nursing documentation tend to be impersonal, usually focusing on completion of the tasks rather than their outcome.

> W/L admission to ward for above surgery tomorrow. TPR and BP ✓ Urinalysis ✓ Weight ✓ Clothes ✓.

In interviews, the admitting nurse would give either an account that focused on the admission and the tasks, or a more personalised account which referred to the patient by name or third person pronoun.

> I carried out the normal admission procedures for nursing staff – so I did blood pressure, pulse, temperature . . .

> Mrs [ ] came in about half past 9–10 o'clock and I took her temperature, introduced her to the ladies in the cubicle and took her temperature and pulse and blood pressure and she gave me a urinalysis and I did her weight . . .

It was common for nurses in both their written notes and in interviews to refer to completion of the admitting procedure in its entirety.

> Nurse: . . . just admitting him, doing normal nursing procedure, normal admission procedure.

> Notes: Fully admitted by nursing staff . . .

The tasks included in the Admitting rite are listed in Table 5.

Completion of the tasks within this rite are given a high priority by nurses. Nurses will strive to complete them during the nursing duty in which the patient is admitted even when they considers themselves to be 'very busy'.

> I admitted him and that's really all I've had to do with him because there's been no time to do anything else.

TABLE 5: Admitting tasks performed by nurses

Type of admission [acute or waiting list]
Time of admission
Recording: Weight
          Urinalysis
          Temperature
          Pulse
          Respiration
          Blood pressure
Ordering of meals
Wristband in place
Bedcard in place
Recording and storage of clothing
Recording and storage of valuables
Entry of patient details in admission book

Nursing judgement is exercised in the way each nurse organises the individual tasks into an integrated procedure. Skill is required to perform each task proficiently and to attain valid readings. Judgement is also apparent in the interpretation of results. In the following example, the nursing response to finding a patient's blood pressure was abnormally high at the time of admission was to note the result in the nursing notes and institute four-hourly monitoring.

> Commenced on 4 hrly BP recordings. BP 160/100 130/100 on admission.

Nursing judgement can also be inferred from the non-recording of findings. Analysis of the data revealed that no abnormal findings discovered during the patient's admission were omitted from the nursing documentation. Thus, nurses were evaluating the results and recording only the noteworthy ones.

While admission is a nursing procedure associated with entry into the Nursing Partnership, it is a rite which primarily supports the work of other hospital staff who will be involved with the patient during hospitalisation. Thus, the nurse's admitting work can be clearly seen to affect the patient's total hospital experience.

Appraising[6]

Within the field data it was possible to identify a second type of work performed by the nurse during the initiation of a patient into the Nursing Partnership. The primary goal is to establish an initial nursing information base on the patient which will be significant in the subsequent nursing of the patient.

Evidence of appraisal can be found in the initial entries in the nursing documentation which records each patient's passage. However, in this study the quantity and quality of the nursing appraisal and its written record were variable, even when a standard documentation format was in existence to guide the activity.

Two variations of the nursing history format were available to the nurses (both forms are present in Appendix 8). However, only five patients from three wards had any formalised nursing history completed. Of these, two were recorded on the form devised specifically for surgical patients and three were written on the alternative form which had been prepared for use in any area of the hospital. Charge nurses in two of the five wards in the study had decided not to use any formal history form and, instead, asked their staff to make a short comment on the patient's social situation in the 'Special Cares' section of the nursing care plan.

Analysis of the data revealed that there had been no planned collection of a nursing database for eight patients, while another eight had minimal social information recorded on the care plan. Of the five nursing histories which were completed, three were filled in by registered nurses and two by student nurses. Members from both groups omitted to complete them.

The history form in general use was primarily a checklist with some open-ended questions. These drew the nurse's attention to selected aspects of the person's normal pattern of daily living as well as the patient's manner during the interview. The history form was closely related to the format for the nursing care plan. Questions were grouped under the headings listed in Table 6.

TABLE 6: Areas for investigation in nursing history

Patient's perception and expectations related to illness
  and hospitalisation
Mobility
Hygiene
Rest and sleep
Elimination
Communication
Nutrition
Social needs
Nurse's observation during interview
Communication patterns [during interview]

These headings reflect the perception of nursing's focus of concern held by the originators of the form.

One nurse spoke of her reason for discarding the nursing history form while actually interviewing one of the patients.

> As I was doing the nursing history I found that it wasn't appropriate to what I wanted to hear because it said so many things like, 'How many times do you wash your hair?' and, 'Do you sleep well?' and things like that. I explained to him that the nursing history was to help me nurse him. So I just sort of discarded that and thought, No, it wasn't appropriate, and I said to him, 'Well, do you know of anything that would help me nurse you better?' to which I got a lovely response . . .

Another nurse justified not using the form in her ward by also questioning the usefulness of the information sought.

We don't use them in this ward. If we ever do, they are just tucked away and never used. What's the use of asking someone how often they shampoo their hair, or how many pillows they sleep with when there's only two on each bed, or whether they like their windows open or shut when we can't open the windows. I can see the reason for doing the social history because that's important, but to find out what their normal life is like at home is of limited use if the information is not available or we can't do anything about it while the person is in hospital.

A charge nurse shared her concern that it was difficult to persuade her staff to consistently complete a nursing history.

Yes, I expect them to do it [history and care plan] but they don't do it . . . . They're not encouraged to use the nursing histories throughout the hospital. They find the forms difficult to use. In reality there's a lot of questions on that form that we ask and we get answers and there's nothing we can do about the answers anyway — questions about ventilation and what their likes and dislikes are. Well, I suppose we can do something about meals and one or two pillows and that sort of thing. I ask them to explain to the patient why we can't do some things, but that would appear to be too much trouble for some people and they don't use the form.

These comments indicate some of the areas of perceived difficulty in using nursing history forms to gather a nursing database during initial appraisal. In particular, nurses seemed to experience difficulty in linking the information obtained in the nursing history to nursing decision-making and action. Thus, the format failed to generate the kind of information that nurses valued and could use during the partnership.

Appraisal involves more than asking questions. Nurses are also establishing a database on each patient while undertaking each activity during the patient's initiation. All information is interpreted by the nurse. In their responses to the question: 'How has Mr [ ] been since he came in and what kind of nursing has he required?', nurses gave an insight into what they considered important. Two examples of replies to this question suggest that nurses give priority to patients' statuses at the time of entering hospital and their readiness for their surgery, rather than their normal pattern of daily living.

Well, she came in about 10 o'clock this morning. She was accompanied by her husband and a friend of hers — a younger female friend. She didn't appear too nervous, really — but as we were talking, once her relatives had gone home and I was admitting her, we had a good talk and I think she was slightly nervous although she seems more worried about social problems – her moving and associated problems, her urinary frequency and things like that – more than she seems worried about having cancer or having a breast removed. She's worried about post-operative pain. We assured her about that and the pain-relief injections that we can give her . . .

I found [   ] very relaxed – ah – very cheerful. She has a very positive outlook about her condition. She didn't seem at all worried about the operation. She was willing to ask questions . . . . I found her a very nice girl . . . and her mother seemed very supportive.

Nurses also seek information on the patients' previous experience of hospitalisation in order to identify the nature and amount of knowledge available to them as they enter into this experience of being nursed.

Well, he's obviously a man who's been in hospital before and is used to the situation. He didn't appear to feel out of place. He sort of knew what he was coming to . . .

Well, he told me it's the first time he's been in hospital for an operation so he's been a bit anxious.

Data such as these last four excerpts became the source for defining the work of both patient and nurse within the Nursing Partnership. Although not guided to do so by the documentation format, nurses were gathering information that showed an interpretation of the patient's situation, albeit an informal and unorganised one, which seemed to override the nursing history. For example, the nurses quoted are speaking of information which can be related to some of the areas of patient work such as: Becoming a Patient, Suspending Social Roles, Managing Self, Surviving the Ordeal and Interpreting the Experience.

However, examination of the nursing notes of the patients referred to above reveals that nurses did not translate this acquired information into a written record. Nor is it present in the notes of the other patients in the study. Indeed, very little of the informal nursing appraisal was transcribed into the nursing record, although these excerpts from interviews reveal its presence. Occasionally it could be deduced from the nursing care plan.

The nursing care plan used in the five wards in this study was consistent with the problem-oriented approach to diagnosis and care planning currently favoured in nursing. A copy of these nursing care plans can be found in Appendix 9. There are two major sections to the form – problems and orders. After appraising the patient using the established criteria, the nurse is requested to deliberate on the results and identify any 'Nursing Problems' – present or anticipated. In the space alongside each problem she enters the 'Nursing Aims' which are considered appropriate to achieve its resolution. The remainder of the two-page care plan requires the writing of nursing orders in relation to specific topics: mental state, nutrition, observations, hygiene, mobility, elimination and special cares. Two extra topics – rest and sleep, and records – are included on the medical nursing care plan, which was used for two subjects.

In a way, this care plan format served as a guide for the appraising activities of the nurse. It assumes that nurses gather information on the status of the client in relation to each topic. The cues are filtered by the nurse and are recorded only if they can be expressed as a problem which is considered to require a planned nursing response.

Table 7 is a representative example of the nursing care plans completed on the patients in this study following the appraising activities of the nurse.

If no problems are noted, as in this case, the care plan consists of a prescription for activities common to all patients – daily bowel check, daily recordings of temperature and pulse – and routine preoperative activities – checklist, nothing by mouth.

Only seven of the 21 patients had any nursing problems identified on the nursing care plan following the initial appraisal. However, problems were identified in the nursing notes of 11 patients, and 11 of the appraising nurses spoke of patient problems during interviews. Lists of the problems identified in each of these three forms of data are presented in Table 8.

Although the study was not designed to evaluate the ability of nurses to recognise, describe and name nursing problems, inconsistencies are evident in the lists compiled from the data. The table reveals variations between the lists in both the problems and the patients. Only one problem – 'loss of memory' – was identified in the nursing notes, nursing care plan and the interview of the same patient. Six problems were identified in the nursing notes and interviews relating to six patients; one problem was noted in the notes and care plan but not the interview; while one was noted in the care plan and interview but not the nursing notes. The remainder were identified in only one form of data.

TABLE 7: Sample nursing care plan completed following initial appraisal

---

Situation – Person admitted with possible recurrence of cancer

Nursing Problems:	Nil
Mental Status:	Alert and oriented
Nutrition:	Normal diet
	NPM [nothing by mouth from] 2400
Observations:	Daily TP [temperature and pulse]
Hygiene:	Shower
Mobility:	Up as able
Elimination:	Daily bowel check
Special Cares:	Preop checklist

The data obtained in this study revealed that the nurses were finding it difficult to establish a nursing database on patients at the point of entry. There is evidence that nurses did not have access to an appraisal protocol which would be consistent with a theoretical intrepretation of the patient's total experience, and which would consistently yield meaningful information relevant to nursing. Despite this, however, the behaviour of the nurses in this study, as reflected in the nursing documentation and interviews, indicates significant appraisal work by the nurse during the initiation of each patient into the Nursing Partnership.

An appraisal format is required that is consistent with the patient and nurse work within the partnership. This would add meaning to the work which nurses are presently doing during the Settling In phase. Their appraisal would be structured in a way that would focus it on the nursing dimensions of the patient's total experience, and would establish an information base which is relevant to nursing's contribution to the patient.

As discussed, the research data revealed that nurses must make appraisals at the patient's point of entry. However, the format in use at the time of the study did not seem to be achieving the desired result of establishing a useful information base on which to base subsequent nursing intervention. Meanwhile it was discovered that patients also have an identifiable pattern of work to do during this initiation experience as they make the transition from home and their usual pattern of daily living to the role of a patient who is about to undergo surgery.

TABLE 8: Nursing problems identified during initial appraisal

In Nursing Care Plans –
  7 patients

Reduced vision (3)
Anxiety (2)
Fear – preoperative
Anxiety and lack of knowledge
Postoperative complications (2)
Pain (2)
Dialysis patient
Back pain due to recent
  kidney infections
Frequency and 'disurea'
  [dysuria]
Loss of memory
Says he forgets easily
Blackouts on occasions
Difficulty sleeping at times

In Nursing Notes –
  11 patients

High blood pressure (2)
Loss of memory
Loose cough
Not sleeping/poor sleep
  pattern (2)
Pain/cramp in leg
Anxiety (2)
Anxiety – pain
Anxiety – surgery
Anxiety – re leg
Apprehension
Smoking
Walks with a stick

In Nurse Interviews –
  – 11 patients

Apprehension (2)
Concern over cancer
Communication problem
Anxiety (2)
Not sleeping/poor sleep
  pattern (3)
Anxiety – home situation
Anxiety – diuretics
Anxiety – pain
Conflict/confusion over
  procedure
Lack of trust in nurses
  concerning dialysis
Loss of memory
Occasional blackouts
Lack of family support
No dentures
Shortness of breath
Worry about ability of
  the surgeon

---

¹ Nurses consistently used the term 'Settling In' to indicate that the patient had completed the process of admission to hospital and into nursing care. A qualitative judgement on the patient's transition was implied in the nurses' use of the term, for example, 'Settling into the ward well', 'Has settled well into the ward'.

[2]   In this context the use of the gerundial 'Becoming' reflects the process of transition experienced by the patient during the period of Settling In. The term 'Patient' was chosen instead of 'client' because that was the terminology used by the patient, the nursing staff, and all others in the institution.

[3]   This term reflects most appropriately what patients were saying. They showed evidence of recognising the need to give up some responsibilities for the duration of the surgery and recovery period. In this context 'Suspending' means 'causing to cease temporarily' (Collins, 1979).

[4]   This term reflects the loss of privacy. 'Revealing' is used to mean 'disclosing; divulging; exposing to view' (Collins, 1979).

[5]   This term was developed from the data itself. It was used by nurses to refer to the set of tasks which they were required to undertake in order to gather initial general data from patients and to settle them into the hospital environment – '. . . just admitting him'.

[6]   'Appraising' describes the nursing work undertaken during the patient's initiation into hospital. 'Appraising' is defined as 'assessing' the distinguishing characteristics, properties or attributes of the patient (Collins, 1979).

5 NEGOTIATING THE NURSING PARTNERSHIP: THE WORK OF THE PATIENT

From the time patients enter hospital and begin their initiation into the Nursing Partnership, they face some of the many internal and external challenges which will continually confront them throughout the passage. This dramatic moment-by-moment negotiation process characterises the patient's passage through the partnership, and provides the focus and purpose for nursing action.

From the interviews with patients as they lived through the experience of hospitalisation and the surgery itself, four distinct areas of patient work could be identified. Firstly, patients had to learn to cope with the experience. Secondly, they had to establish a relationship with the various helping people. Thirdly, each patient had to try to get through the potentially threatening experience of having a disease process which required medical intervention in the form of surgery, anaesthetic and the aftermath. Finally, the patient was constantly receiving and analysing information, synthesising data, and translating this interpretation into a personally meaningful account of the ongoing experience.

Although the existence of these four areas of patient activity became evident quite early during the data collection and analysis, they were not confirmed as being the most useful perspective on nursing-relevant patient behaviour until many alternatives had been attempted and discarded. The compilation of this model of patient behaviour was a lengthy process despite the consistency in the ideas contained in the many diary notes, analytical notations written in the data, and the theoretical memos.

The data was analysed to see if the problem which surfaced for the patient during the Beginning phase of the passage was the most significant pattern around which patients organised their behaviour. This did not prove to be a valid basis for distinction between patients' behaviour although the nature of the problem helped shape patient behaviour within the four constructs of the model's final form. It is possible that further research on the

patient's passage within the Nursing Partnership will link negotiation work with the impact of the health problem itself.

Throughout the Nursing Partnership the patients can be seen
to be working on their total situation. This work is relevant to
nursing because the nurse has the mandate, knowledge and skills to
share this experience with the patient, giving specialised assistance
to help the patient in this work. Thus, nursing has a pivotal role in a
patient's hospitalisation and, in this study, surgery.

Four concepts identify the different areas in which patients
negotiate their way through the Nursing Partnership: Managing
Self, Affiliating with Experts, Surviving the Ordeal, and Interpreting the Experience. A summary of these complex constructs
together with their subconcepts is presented in Table 9.

TABLE 9: Negotiating the Nursing Partnership: the work of
the patient

Managing Self	Affiliating with Experts
Centring on Self	Acquiescing to Expertise
Harnessing Resources	Fitting In
Maintaining Equanimity	Retaining Autonomy
Surviving the Ordeal	Interpreting the Experience
Enduring Hardship	Developing Expertise
Tolerating Uncertainty	Monitoring Events
Possessing Hope	

Although each concept is discussed as a discrete entity, each concept influences and is influenced by the others. Thus, the patient's
behaviour is a complex and integrated network of these activities.

It may also seem that the goals suggested by each construct are
attainable, and indeed have been attained, by the individual efforts
of each patient. This is not the case. Success alone or within the
specialised partnership with the nurse, is not guaranteed. Perhaps
it rarely occurs. Rather, the data suggested that patients are continually working in each of these areas throughout the passage.
Nursing works with patients to try to achieve the best results within
the reality of their situation.

To date, the Nursing Partnership has not been developed to
the stage where areas of patient and nurse work can be linked to
hypothesised patient outcomes. Further research would be required

to accomplish this. Within the present data, however, both patient and nurse can be seen to be working together to progress the patient through the passage, although no definitive criteria for success, in either patient or nursing terms, have been defined.

Managing Self[1]

In the Beginning, the patient's preparation for admission to hospital for elective surgery was discussed. As the anticipation becomes reality, patients pay considerable attention to themselves and the way they will cope with the anticipated challenge. Patients bring with them the self-management practices that have already been learned. While these are the key factors in a patient's ability to cope with the events, they are modified by the meaning the person attaches to the problem and their perception of appropriate patient behaviour. The actions and reactions of staff and others are influential in this.

Another aspect of managing self which became apparent in the data was the patient's acceptance of the contribution of personal responsibility to the outcome of the surgery.

> My priorities are to make sure I do my bit to make sure this works out because [the surgeon] has done his bit and the nurse can put drops in it. I think the main thing is my own action – not being stupid over the thing, not bending down or jerking or getting out of bed and roaming around the ward.

One patient described her responsibilities as:

> Have the right attitude, be optimistic and do all I can for myself.

She went on to state:

> I'll try as hard as I possibly can at everything and, even if I can't do it, the nurses should know I've done my best. But, I'll need quite a bit of help from them.

Three significant dimensions in the patient's management of self emerged as subconcepts: Centring on Self, Harnessing Resources, and Maintaining Equanimity. These concepts specify the range of patient activities which help patients' self-management as it applies to being nursed while undergoing surgery.

Centring on Self[2]: The whole environment, including the behaviour of the people within the hospital setting, encourages the patient to focus on self. The presenting problem, the patient's body and personal health-related information are exposed for examination by experts.

> If you didn't have anything wrong with you before, you certainly would have by the time they had done their checks!

Patients are constantly asked how they are feeling.

> There's lots of people been coming in and asking me if I was alright.

The patient, or the problem requiring surgery, is the centre of attention during visits by medical and nursing staff.

> [The doctors] didn't do much. They just showed the young students the foot where the melanoma was. Seems to be the drawcard for everyone to have a look. I am having a collection box here! A dollar a look!

In addition patients' attention is forced onto themselves as the impact of the problem and its therapy are felt.

> I sat on a plank, you know, across the bath, and splashed all over, and that was very nice. Then I came back and I felt very, very tired and I felt more sore than usual. My wounds were desperately sore – sorer than any other time. My back was tired and, of course, I have this disc trouble. And I couldn't find a comfortable place for my back and I just felt more and more miserable.

This centring on self can be considered as a conservation strategy as well as a consequence of the situation. It focuses the patient's energies on the challenge and attaining the best results.

> When you're not well, you know, you've got to look after yourself.

In one interview the patient confirmed his awareness of this self-centredness but he also went on to express concern about such behaviour.

> I'm getting conceited because all I'm thinking about is myself.

However, this behaviour is validated by social sanction. Encouragement is given by hospital staff, family and friends for the patient to suspend usual social roles and responsibilities for the duration of the experience.

Harnessing Resources[3]: In order to manage the experience, each patient draws on strategies that have previously been developed to meet the challenges of daily life. Patients identify what they believe they need to do to endure the present experience and to maximise the chances of success.

> Everything's just floating along. It's just waiting for that healing stage which you can't hurry. You've got to have patience and tolerance and perseverance and all the other things.

Many patients linked the amount of rest and sleep they were able to get to their ability to handle a stressful situation.

> I adapt pretty quickly. As long as you can have a few hours decent sleep you are alright.

> If you have a good night's sleep you don't feel your pains and things do you?

Some patients manage the effects of the surgery itself by appearing to value, even welcome, it as a way of confronting the threatening presence of cancer. If surgery is possible, then there is hope! One patient shared how she coped in this way, and distinguished between this and how she might have regarded surgery in the absence of malignancy.

> I mean I didn't really mind going through the operation if the result was going to be okay. That was the part that was worrying me. Mind you, if it had been a gallbladder operation, I'd have been worried about it from the word go – about the operation itself. But in this case it seemed to be a secondary thing, having to put up with it.

The patient's strategies may be unrealistic in the long-term but may be the best way of coping in the immediate circumstances. For example, several patients spoke of avoiding seeing the wound at the time of the first dressing change. However, others may feel able to look at the healing wound.

> It's all exposed now . . . . And, anyway, I was just thanking him [surgeon] and I was saying I was quite surprised at the end result. 'Ooh,' he said, 'The end result hasn't arrived yet.' I don't know what he meant by that . . . . This [mastectomy suture line] looks nothing, but the part under there [at side] didn't look nice when I saw myself in the bathroom – to me who's not used to wounds.

> [The nurse] insisted in getting a mirror to show me what a wonderful job it was but I wasn't really interested. I might sound slightly squeamish. I still haven't seen it but I'm not in a hurry to.

Coping mechanisms are effective when they are balanced with, or superior to, the challenge facing the person. There seems little doubt that reflection beforehand permits patients to prepare themselves as far as possible for what they believe lies ahead.

> Not worrying – just the fact that I'll be having to adjust my eyes and may or may not be able to drive and am still having to get this dialysis going. I think that's a fairly good handful for me to handle. It won't get me down but it's enough.

The nurse may need to do a variety of things to supplement the patient's personal resources. Indeed, often the patient cannot manage alone. Many aspects of nursing's work within the Nursing Partnership assist the patient by providing external, supplementary energy. Examples of this are easily found. They include such practical actions as the selective administration of pain relief, making the patient comfortable, giving information that is appropriate in timing, language and amount, and being present to give confidence.

Even seemingly mundane assistance is valued. For example, one patient's position in the bed was making it hard, indeed almost impossible, to manage eating a meal. The nurse researcher adjusted her position, altered the pillows and also secured the meal tray.

> Oh that's given me support. Ooh, that's lovely. Now I can cope with two hands. I was really cock-eyed.

Maintaining Equanimity[4]: During the Beginning, the person has worked at achieving a state of personal equanimity or composure to the circumstances of the upcoming surgery. Entry into hospital changes the situation from anticipation to reality, and the work continues. Now the patient is actually in the hospital and the time for the surgery is at hand. Indeed, patients increasingly feel its impact within themselves and in the actions of the hospital staff.

One patient, whose surgery had complications, revealed after discharge that he had become very uncertain about his agreement to the surgery soon after admission because the surgeon revealed new information during his examination.

> It came as a bit of a surprise to me when I saw him in hospital before the operation, the very day before, when he explained about this vision [postoperative problem to adjust vision in two eyes] and that night I didn't sleep too well. I thought about it quite a bit and thought 'Am I doing the right thing?' . . . I am not critical of it at all.

Comments such as this reveal the tenuousness of the assent and the hidden confusion and/or uncertainty which may be going on in a patient who, on the surface, appears composed and acquiescent. New or conflicting information may challenge the patient's equanimity throughout the duration of the passage. Within the partnership, appropriate nursing action can bring real benefit.

The environment itself may cause a degree of apprehension as the patient enters the hospital.

> I do have a bit of apprehension coming in this morning. The initial thing you strike is car parking . . . . and it was raining . . . Then when we came through the front entry, it's a rather forbidding place. I would imagine some people could get quite upset by it – if they were the worried or nervous types . . . . But once the cubbyhole was opened – very friendly – no problems.

In spite of challenges to their equanimity, the patients in this study gave the impression that they were continually striving to maintain their self-control as the time for the actual surgery drew nearer.

> I am anxious about tomorrow but I am not. I won't lose any sleep over it. I'll be glad to get it done.

> I'm alright now. Now I know it's going to happen.

> So we'll do our best and we'll just cross our fingers and hope.

It is difficult to transmit the quality of composure by the words used alone. The context of the conversation, the manner of speaking and the dignity demonstrated by these patients as they recounted their experience conveyed a sense of quietude and order. Perhaps the argument for this patient state is enhanced by further reference to the one patient, mentioned in Chapter 3, who had not attained it by the time she was admitted.

> . . . when I came here this morning I just freaked out . . . . I just felt so uptight. Uptight is probably the understatement of the century. Total anxiety! . . . . I was pretty anxious. The nurse that I met was really nice and put me at ease and I was able to talk. I had to talk to somebody. Both the charge nurse and the student nurse. They were just great – really nice people and I felt immediately better and they told me to ask the surgeon when he came round, to ask questions because I knew so little. But when he comes round with a cast of ten around the bed you don't actually get around to saying anything. You sort of coy out on him. But I feel a lot more relaxed now than I did when I walked through that door this morning.

Her disquiet became evident to the appraising nurse, a student, who shared her concern with the charge nurse. The latter recounted the situation.

> There's nothing wrong with her. She was going to Mr [   ] and, when he got sick, she had to switch to Mr [   ]. She had a bad time with the old registrar in clinic. I had a chat with her and told her to ask Mr [   ] when he came round but when he got to the bed he said, 'I understand you want to ask me something.' She was a bit put off by this and couldn't get her questions out. I'll have to go back and speak with her but she's alright.

Through her nursing actions, the charge nurse was able to provide the additional resources essential to allow the patient to attain and maintain equanimity. By the following day, while waiting to go to theatre, the patient's words and manner confirmed her relative serenity.

> When I saw you yesterday I probably was a bit uptight. Of course I will be pleased when it's all over.

Humour was often present in the interviews conducted soon after admission. The focus of the joking was often something outside the control of the patient. Indeed, such humour, often black, may be one way of maintaining self-control in a potentially frightening situation. In the following examples, humour is used in references to the length of the surgeon's operating day, the preparation of the operating list, the skill of nurses and the anaesthetic. These are all issues within the domain of the experts on whom the patient is now dependent.

> Imagine operating all day! I certainly wouldn't like to be at the end of the day if he was. 'Oh, who's this one? Arm? Leg?'

> Nice nurse. She was very gentle. I thought I might strike a rough one! [Laughs]

> I know I'm getting slotted in somewhere. I think I must be the preliminary warm-up! [Name was not on operation list]

> I don't mind once I'm out to it what happens! [Laughs] I'm glad I didn't live a few years ago when you had to bite a rag or something!

Throughout the Nursing Partnership, the patient is constantly challenged by new experiences which include pain, sleeplessness, discomfort, waiting, enforced immobility, and uncertainty. During each stage the patient strives to maintain composure.

> I think I've got the kind of nature that, when a thing happens, I accept it. You know, when you can't fight against it, go with it.

> When it [pain] comes on, I think about it, then it goes off and it's alright again. I stay quiet.

During the time in hospital patients may receive news which could have a profound effect on their future. In the following example, the patient describes his reaction to being confronted with the news that the surgery had failed and it was possible, even probable, that his leg would need to be amputated.

> When they started talking about taking the leg off and things, I didn't fly into a panic or anything like that, but it takes a bit of absorbing, you know.

Later he spoke of the way in which he sought to maintain his composure during the remainder of the day, including the impact of his reaction on other events.

> That's been my day really, trying to put this at the back of my mind and, of course, getting uptight with the nurse. I didn't say anything to her. I would never do that. It was probably me being upset and I didn't say anything to her. I just went along with it.

This example suggests that patients consider their efforts to maintain equanimity successful if they achieve a composed exterior despite a degree of turmoil inside. Thus, patients try to conceal feelings which are considered to be inappropriate in the circumstances.

> I was very nervous [before surgery] but I tried to hide it. It was nerve-wracking to think about it.

Such behaviour presents a real challenge to nurses as they seek to ease the patient through the passage. Identifying areas of turmoil without damaging the patient's attempts to maintain composure requires considerable nursing skill.

Sometimes efforts to maintain equanimity are reinforced by paying attention to the ways in which patients presents themselves to the world. For women, continuing activities such as the use of make-up and care of the hair may increase the feeling of composure and self-control.

> I was just going to comb my hair and put my lipstick on and try to look brighter.

Achieving equanimity in the presence of considerable discomfort may be helped if the state has been predicted and adequately explained beforehand by an expert. In the following example the expert was the physician who had referred the patient for surgery.

> I feel so weak. I've got no energy whatsoever. [   ] told me I would feel like this. I would feel absolutely dreadful for a couple of days and my calcium would go all to pot and down, but they would gradually start building it up and I would gradually start feeling better. And I do really feel dreadful. But that's what I expected.

However, no patient can be totally prepared beforehand for an experience that has not been previously encountered. Within the Nursing Partnership, the patient is able to benefit from the individual nurses who seek to ease the patient through unexpected as well as anticipated events.

The number and type of unexpected challenges to equanimity which may be encountered during time in hospital varies between patients. These often arise from the medical equipment, such as an intravenous infusion becoming detached during the night and/or multiple attempts by inexperienced medical staff to insert a needle to restart an infusion – a common feature in the data.

> It was about 10.30. I woke up and I could feel something damp on my arm and it was my life blood flowing out. They had to change the bed and everything . . . . I think I had used the bottle and when I put it back I think I got the cord jammed in it with the result when I moved on to my side, I pulled it and it just broke . . . . They didn't have to replace the whole thing. They soon had it back to normal.

However, it was evident the infusion was flowing poorly and would soon need to be replaced. The following afternoon this man had another story to tell.

> I suppose it was about half past 6 when they finished. It took two doctors and five needles before they did . . . . I'll give the first doctor his due. He did it up here [pointing to elbow area] and it's the first time anyone has put a painkiller there first. It was only a prick in comparison to the other needles. When he didn't get a result, he said, 'I'm not going to do any more.' I presume by that he is fairly new at it . . . . He went away and rang someone up. So then she proceeded to have her go. She went there and got no result, so she went there and got no result. I thought 'Gee, I hope you get a result soon. I'm running out of spots!'

In addition, in the life-and-death setting of the hospital where many patients are facing personal crises, tragic events do occur and these affect those who share the environment. The following comments from two patients reflect the way in which both were seeking to maintain their composure as they reacted to the sudden death of a patient in the same room.

> It didn't bother me. It's one of those things. It's got to happen. You won't go before your time. When your time is up, you'll go no matter what you do. I'm fatalistic in that respect.

> You probably found out we had a bit of a problem this morning. I went out in the other room and had breakfast in the other room. Didn't find out till later that he had gone. Stuns you a bit!

As previously stated, equanimity is not always possible by the efforts of the patient alone. Indeed, from time to time a patient may falter and feel overwhelmed by the situation. Nurses are often granted the privilege of hearing a patient admit this, or of identifying cues that indicate this. Comments such as the following are cues that suggest the patient will welcome nursing assistance to help restore a state of peace.

> I am really a bit confused just now. I don't know whether I am coming or going.

Affiliating with Experts[5]

A person enters hospital in order to receive the specialised assistance necessary to resolve a health problem. This help is given through the services of a variety of health professions – nursing, medicine, physiotherapy, occupational therapy, radiography and many more. Additional help comes from other groups who contribute to the daily maintenance of the hospital and its services – cleaning, kitchen, clerical, porter and others. Many representatives of these groups come into personal contact with the patient. Some meet the patient on only one occasion; others come into relationships which last throughout the person's stay.

From the patient's perspective, there is the job of identifying each face by group, by title and, perhaps, by name. Then there is the task of clarifying the specific nature of the service offered – each group, each visit, each person. Patients quickly learn that there are individual differences in the approaches and the expertise of the people they encounter. Wisdom grew within the patients in this study as their personal experience of each group and each individual helper increased.

There is work for the patients to do as they enter into associations of varying closeness and importance with each person and each group. There is an awareness that there will be times when, following submission, they are totally under the control of other people, as happens, for example, when a person is unconscious during surgery. There seems no doubt that patients try to cooperate as much as possible with the experts in order to obtain the best resolution of the problem. However, for most of the time, patients seem to retain some autonomy over themselves and to exercise some selectivity in the degree to which they accede to orders, advice or rules.

Three subconcepts within this major construct have been identified: Acquiescing to Expertise, Fitting In, and Retaining Autonomy. Each reflects a different dimension of the independence/dependence dichotomy in patients' relationships with the various groups of specialist hospital staff.

Acquiescing to Expertise[6]: This aspect has previously been referred to during the discussion on both the Beginning and Settling In. Now it emerges as a significant and separate concept. As in the previous phases, the patient is prepared to follow instructions from the experts – particularly medical and nursing personnel – because these are considered to arise from their specialised knowledge.

> I've been allowed to take my pad off today so that's the big event.

> Look what I've got to do now all the time [breathing exercises].

> Apparently I've got to go and have a shower first.

> If I want to go to the toilet, I have to go and see them [nurses] again.

Undoubtedly, there is a degree of submission present in the acquiescence of patients. However, it seems to be most willingly given when there is confidence and trust in the person and the reason for the request.

> I want to get out and have a bath or shower but I can't until the doctor says.

> He wanted me to have bedrest, not to be getting up or trying to walk or anything like that.

Even when the prescribed treatment is not pleasant, or the patient would have made a different decision if given the opportunity, the patient attempts to adhere to the regimen prescribed by the expert. The course of action is presumed to be beneficial.

> I've been drinking. I've nearly drowned in water. I've just about drunk the sea dry, I think. And then they brought me those pills and there's quite a lot of them. I said I'd be rattling very soon. They're two every hour.

> I think I could actually have gone home today, I felt, but he said tomorrow and I won't argue with him.

Acquiescing may be associated with a sense of powerlessness in the presence of the expert person, particularly the surgeon. The power of the surgeons is significant because of the work they do and is further increased by the reliance placed on their short and often irregular visits for major decisions concerning care, outcome of surgery and discharge. Authority and trust are ascribed to them, and many patients are passive in the surgeon's presence.

> Yesterday he [the surgeon] came. He seemed to be quite satisfied. Holding my hand. You don't get much satisfaction. I suppose they will talk to you before you leave or you can go and see them, can't you . . . . You do [have the opportunity to ask questions] but what could I ask him? Only what I keep thinking about − that I hope I won't have any more trouble. I suppose he gets that all the time and gets sick of being asked.

> Not long ago Mr [   ] came round and I was getting up on my feet. I was going for a walk along the passage. He said, 'You could just about have that [nasogastric tube] out.' He said, 'What have you been getting out of that today, Nurse?' And she told him and he said, 'I'll tell you what, as long as you don't drink anything but ice, you can have it out.' I said, 'It's a deal.' He said, 'Right, take it out.'

Deference is not so apparent in the relationships with nurses in which contact is more frequent, as assistance is given in the moment-by-moment activities of the patient's passage.

> Nurse gave me a pain relief before she got me up for a wash and that. She sat me up there. She found a sheepskin for me. So she put that on . . . . I had a bit of pain at the bottom of my tummy. I thought it might be because my bowels haven't moved since I came in. She gave me a suppository and I sat there for two hours . . . . She said to have a tablet tonight because I am used to going every morning . . . . I sat out while they made the bed . . . . Nurse said my

bottom wasn't red or anything and she gave me a little bit of a rub there.

This different relationship is significant for nursing. It gives the nurse an opportunity to work more closely than any other group on a personal basis with patients as they react to the consequences of reliance on the expertise of others. For example, the deference ascribed to the senior medical staff, together with their pattern of intermittent visiting, which is often associated with critical decision-making, may generate feelings of uncertainty, even fear. Supportive activities, such as filling in the gaps or transcribing medical terminology into everyday English after a doctor's visit, may be required from the nurse. The nurse can also help by ascertaining the patient's areas of concern prior to medical visits and encouraging the patient to express these, or even conveying these to the medical staff on the patient's behalf.

Fitting In[7]: Fitting In is a concept developed to reflect the adaptation, or sense of belonging, the patient attempts to achieve in relation to the people, the system and the hospital environment. It indicates that patients sense a need to 'fit in' because they feel an obligation to the staff. Staff members are there to help that person and the other patients in the ward.

> [The staff nurse] asked me if I'd like a bath. This was before morning tea. I said, 'Does it make any difference when I have my bath?' I mean, I wanted to fit in with her. She said, 'No, I can give it to you now or before lunch, whichever you prefer.

Seeing the nursing staff as partners in a joint endeavour allows the patient to feel involved in the experience. Thus, fitting in can also include a sense of alliance with the nurse to ensure treatments, procedures, and so forth, are carried out.

> Doctors came around and wondered why the stocking hadn't been put on yesterday. So [the staff nurse] rushed around and put it on. I had forgotten about it myself or I would have reminded them. Poor [staff nurse].

This sense of joint responsibility extends to the patient becoming familiar with what will indicate progress and maintaining a sensitivity to its occurrence. As in the following example, normal daily activities assume importance, and even generate excitement, when they are perceived to be indicators of progress.

> I had that beautiful bowel movement today. I am proud of that. Mr
> [   ] laid stress on that. He said as far as he is concerned its a sign that
> everything is working after the operation and this is what they look
> for to find out.

The mutual geniality which is commonly found in the partnership
between patients and nurses reflects the cooperation which the
patient seeks to maintain.

> Well, I make it as pleasant as I can for them and they make it as
> pleasant as they can for me.

Even practices which are perceived to border on the absurd are
accepted with good humour and even, occasionally, as in the following example from a patient interview, with a touch of sarcasm.

> . . . and next thing it was the 6 o'clock ritual of the hospital. You've
> got to wake them at 6 o'clock or the world comes to an end! And then
> they go back and relax until 9!

The concept of Fitting In acknowledges the patients' willingness to
change their normal expectations within the hospital environment.
It includes the realisation that the conditions which one has control
over at home − including noise, visitors, light, daily schedule of
personal activities − are not controllable in the hospital ward. This is
particularly apparent in relation to activities such as sleep, food and
hygiene. Patients in this study seemed to be very tolerant in
relation to such issues.

> I had a good night's sleep . . . . There was some toing and froing. It
> must have been about 1 or 2 o'clock in the morning − perhaps earlier
> than that. I think there was an admission or there was somebody
> being difficult in the next ward.

> We had rather a nice lunch − lambs' tongues in mushroom gravy. It
> was tasty. I was a bit frightened to risk it but I tried it and it was
> lovely. Not that crazy on mushrooms but it was alright. Nice baked
> custard too.

Retaining Autonomy[8]: Paradoxically, with the desire to accept the
advice of experts and to adapt to the environment, the patients in
this study consistently demonstrated their retention of a degree of
personal freedom. They revealed this autonomy in a variety of ways.
Sometimes it was apparent in areas outside the immediate health
problem and its therapeutic regime; sometimes it related to general
aspects of the person's experience as a patient; and, on some

occasions, it was linked to the therapy itself. This independence could be either overt or concealed from others. Also, it could remain as independence of thought or extend to autonomous action.

Independent behaviour on the part of patients was rarely confrontational, angry or acrimonious. Only one instance of direct confrontation was recorded in the data when a patient verbally challenged the behaviour of a staff member, in this case the surgeon. According to the patient's perception of the incident, the surgeon only wanted to inspect the wound because the plaster was not adhering to the skin in one place. This patient had been loosening the plaster herself as she had heard from 'somebody' that she would have half of the clips removed from the wound later that day. When he came around, the surgeon reprimanded her for this action.

> I can't believe it. The stupid old – I didn't say that! Most unusual man! I'm told he is conservative in his views. I was upset because the healing process is now stalled somewhat . . . . The plaster was half off so he thought, 'Oh well, I'll have a look,' but I wouldn't let him. It's been a disaster all round, really!

Patients in this study gave no indications of a perceived power conflict with medical or nursing staff. Instead, there was a matter-of-factness in the patients' behaviour which seemed more indicative of a sense of shared control rather than a feeling of total subordination.

In the interviews there are many examples of patients speaking of being offered an opportunity to make a decision by the nurse and their choosing to do so.

> I had a sleeping pill – only one. A little one. I said, 'I'll take one.' 'Take two,' she said. I said, 'No, one will do.'

> So she came and I said, 'Oh I might need one [sedative].' So she gave me one.

> They asked me if I wanted a sleeping pill but I don't believe in them.

> This morning they would have given me lemon drink if I had wanted but I said I preferred the water. Tomorrow I might go on to something else.

However, autonomous behaviour may be deliberately concealed as illustrated by the behaviour of one patient who had been prescribed a small dose of valium three times a day soon after admission.

> I think maybe when I came in they might have thought I was a bit – I don't know if 'nervy' is the right word or not – 'het up', perhaps, about what was happening. But I don't think I was actually.

She commented on the inconsistent administration of the drug.

> Once or twice I've said I don't want it and they've taken it away from me. Once or twice they haven't come at all. They were chopping and changing quite a lot. It must be written down somewhere and some obey it and some don't – or some know my feelings and some don't. But, anyway, I don't mind taking it at night because I don't sleep at night.

And then went on to state:

> I've got two actually, stuck in there [locker] that I haven't taken. I thought if they gave me nothing to take home I might take one at night [laughs] at home for a night or two. I shouldn't be telling you this, should I!

There were occasions when patients, even when aware of what they 'should' be doing, chose not to do as requested.

> I was supposed to wait for a nurse to come around and help me, but I just thought, 'Oh, I can brave the course. I can do it.'

Another patient found it difficult to accept the different regimen of care followed by the present ward team in comparison to his previous experience of the same surgery when the ritual of care had been rigorous and strict. He retained his ability to judge and reach an independent decision despite his overt cooperation.

> I still don't think inwardly that the relaxed system is the right system. I don't sort of agree at this stage . . . . It takes a bit of accepting. While I don't accept it, I'm not critical of it.

However, he went on to indicate that his overt compliance was limited because of his faith in the previous regimen. Indeed, even his present behaviour concealed autonomous decision-making.

> People have different systems, different techniques, fair enough, but my lying quiet, quieter than I have to under this particular system, isn't hurting the system. And, if they said I could get up and jump around and do a dance and make a lot of movement, well, there I would be fighting it. I don't think I would accept it readily.

Some patients seemed to be aware that they could retain a measure of autonomy through deliberately concealing information that could provoke an undesirable response from staff.

I'd like to drink a lot more but I can't. I've drunk more today than I should have. Not that I'd let on!

I don't want to tell them here [about the constipation] because I don't want them to start giving me pills and things to make it work. I don't want that.

However, many patients are also exercising autonomy when they make the decision to seek assistance from the nursing staff.

And I haven't had my bowels moved. I'm going to ask them for a pill. I'll perhaps have one tomorrow morning at breakfast time.

As has already been noted, when people undergo surgery they follow a dynamic path in relation to independence and self-care. At the actual time of surgery they are in a significant state of dependency. As the period of recovery lengthens, there is a gradual withdrawing of nursing presence and a resumption of self-care. In this period of transition there is potential for uncertainty on the part of the patient as the nurse no longer appears to perform, or even offer assistance with, tasks such as those associated with daily hygiene care. Now the initiative is handed back to the patients as they are expected to resume more and more independence.

I'll just go along and have a bath in the bathroom. This bed bath is not necessary any more, I don't think. I'll get in there and get organised.

I had a good wash up and down. They didn't say anything so I just washed up and down myself. I went by myself.

In this study, it seemed that the patients never totally submitted to the experts beyond their conscious decision to accept the surgical procedure. However, they were selective in the people with whom they shared this information. Their proven willingness to retain a degree of autonomy in thought and action seemed to be of value as they tended, and were required, to respond with alacrity to the cues that increased self-care was now appropriate.

Well, it's been very pleasant because I've been allowed up and to do what I flipping well like. I was able to start the day off in the the normal fashion by heading for the bathroom in my own time, and going through all the motions in my own time. It's starting to get a bit of independence back, I think. You feel useless and helpless.

Surviving the Ordeal[9]

Undergoing surgery is an ordeal, although the effect varies considerably between patients. This variation is determined as much by the individual resources available to the person as it is by the significance and the severity of the ordeal itself. In this concept, the emphasis is on the different dimensions associated with the work of survival. Three different subconcepts were identified within the data: Enduring Hardship, Tolerating Uncertainty, and Possessing Hope.

Enduring Hardship[10]: Hardship is associated with a variety of feelings and reactions which are linked in some way to the problem, the surgery and/or being in hospital. Enduring such symptoms seems to be accepted by patients as a part of the experience. Assistance is on hand from both nursing and medical activity. However, this study revealed that patients are prepared to 'put up with' hardship with the expectation that it is a temporary phenomenon.

Each patient's story of endurance is different. The variation is evident in the following excerpts from patients' reflections on their status during an interview.

> Now and again I get a sort of muscular spasm or something. It really goes through!

> Just before lunch I felt a bit funny. I was sitting out in the dayroom and felt almost faint, you know. Still feel a bit wonky.

> I've been feeling alright actually. Only thing is I noticed every time I closed my eyes I see all sorts of figures. I hallucinate a lot for some reason. I don't know what that is. Open my eyes to see something out there and there is nothing there.

> Sweating here and my legs as cold as anything today.

> My back's pretty achey.

> I've got a terrible headache.

> My mouth is so dry. Very sore throat. I'm feeling very sorry for myself.

> Generally washed out. No energy. No desire to do anything.

> I haven't been so good today . . . . My neck has been hurting very much and I have been trying to pass water. Haven't been able to.

Some of the discomfort was linked to the actions of others involved in the care of the patient.

> Dreadful. I've got too much fluid on board . . . . I've never felt so dreadful for a long time. [Too much intravenous fluid]

> Nurse came and took the sutures out this morning. I was holding on to the bed but it wasn't too bad. Just a couple of pulls.

One of the findings in this study was the ways in which patients seemed to have prepared themselves to experience pain during the 24–48 hours after surgery. Most, but not all, seemed to associate their feeling with discomfort rather than intolerable pain.

> If I sort of move it [the eye] around, it can ache a bit. It's got a suggestion of a little bit of stinging . . . certainly nothing uncomfortable that I can't tolerate . . . . You'd think it would be a lot worse.

> I've been fairly good today. I've had no pain, no trouble, so I've got nothing to complain about . . . . I thoroughly enjoyed the day.

> I don't think it's necessary to take a pill. I can grin and bear quite a lot . . . . I know I don't have to but I don't want to be taking drugs. I don't actually agree with it if I can do without it . . . . I'm not in agony with it.

> No, not much pain. Will it get worse?

> Very bad [pain] when I cough or move. Is still a bit sore [after injection].

However, it is possible for patients to reach the end of their ability to endure, even when supported by the work of the nursing staff. This was not a common occurrence in this study. In the following example, the patient became so distressed by the pain and discomfort caused by the suture holding the haemovac tube that he demanded its removal before he would go to sleep. The nursing staff met his demand after a telephone consultation with the house surgeon.

> It hurts like hell. It's pulling in the corners. I think I'll go to sleep when it's out. It's really sore. It really is sore!

Tolerating Uncertainty[11]: Each experience of surgery and a general anaesthetic contains an element of uncertainty before the event, no matter how many previous operations or admissions to hospital there might have been. The patient needs to live with this uncertainty until it is resolved, although it can be minimised by the mutual work of patient and nurse through all stages of the Nursing Partnership.

Even if patients are given preoperative information on what is going to happen, they cannot be knowledgeable about every minute or circumstance of the experience beforehand.

> I don't know what it's going to be like so it's an unknown factor. Of course, I'll be pleased when it's all over.

> I didn't realise what it was going to be.

Sometimes uncertainty before an event is increased by the receipt of conflicting information from members of the staff. In such circumstances, unless the nature of the conflict is known and resolved, the patient can experience confusion as well as lack of certainty. This poses a threat to the trust required to achieve a good working partnership between nurse and patient.

> [The surgeon] said I could get out of bed and then the male nurse said I couldn't. So!

A significant cause of uncertainty is the patient's realisation that decisions are sometimes made, even in the patient's presence, without any direct involvement. The decision-making conversation may take place at the foot of the bed and the patient may hear or not hear, understand or not understand what is being discussed.

> I saw them [doctors] at a distance [end of bed] and they said nothing. They hardly said a thing . . . . No, I'm not actually sure what is going on for the simple reason that this [catheter] was supposed to come out on Friday. That's what the doctor said – one of them. And then I think it may be because there's been a clot of blood come down since.

> I heard him saying something to the sister this morning but often when they are talking you don't fully comprehend what they are talking about. I presume it will be another couple of days like this.

The presence of cancer introduces a long-term uncertainty into the life of a person. Despite this, the patient seems to find strategies to help endure the situation.

> I think we all get the fear of death when anyone tells us we've got cancer anywhere. And cancer of the breast comes as an awful shock because, you know, it usually comes with no warning. And in my case, I just have a tremendous feeling of relief that it hasn't been as bad as I thought it was going to be.

Laboratory examination of tissue removed during the surgery gives further information on the cancer and the result may be available while the patient is still in hospital. This happened with several patients in this study and one was informed her future was very uncertain.

> He made a special trip up here and told me all about that – that it was a cancer tumour in my groin caused from that melanoma – and he said from what they knew they had got everything. But he said you cannot guarantee that it could affect somewhere else. He said that they were going to keep close checks on me. He said the only thing they wouldn't like is for it to get into the blood stream because it can travel and you can't pick it up as quickly.

For other patients, however, the outcome may remove uncertainty.

> I got the path report today and that is good. He [the surgeon] was very matter of fact – 'Good! Fine! Clear! No problems. Appointment in January. See you.'

Possessing Hope[12]: Patients undergoing surgery seem able to visualise a future in which there will be an improvement in their condition. This hope, when supported by encouragement from nursing and medical staff as well as the family, sustains patients through their present circumstances. The future which is anticipated may be minutes or hours away, or it could be days, weeks or longer.

> Oh, it's a bit sore but it's getting, you know, every hour now I think it's getting better now.

> I feel a little washed out. Its going to take a day or two to get rid of the dope they put into you to put you out.

> My one thought is to get through today. That's why I think I'll be better tomorrow if I can just get through today.

> I figure it will take a week before I come right. I might go home by Saturday or Sunday.

> This time next week I'll be back to normal.

Hope is tempered by reality and seems to be consistent with the patient's circumstances. Loneliness, grieving, ageing associated with disability or chronic illness, family concerns, job stress – all were present in the patients in this study as well as the concerns related to the presenting health problem. Despite these, or perhaps because of these, the belief in a favourable future seemed to be a source of support as the patient endured the present.

Patients who face a personal crisis as a result of a problem which has necessitated surgery have a specific hope that the threat has, indeed, been removed.

> I hope it is all over. I don't want any more trouble. Hope it's all gone.

Those patients who are waiting for pathology reports may reveal that consideration of dying is present in their thinking. Even this may be associated with an element of hoping in terms of the future if the news is bad.

> Cancer is a nasty thing. I asked [the surgeon] about the checking of cancer and he said he hadn't had the pathological report on the tests made as yet. I will have the joy or otherwise of knowing later on whether I have it or not. One thing, I'm not going through this again. Not worth it! Anyway, I've had a fair lash over the years. What worries me is the suddenness of it. I want to get a few days' notice so that I can make arrangements.

Hope is a dynamic feeling which is also present in the less dramatic but still significant moments of the patient's experience.

> I have taken a sleeping pill. Hope for the best.

As patients regain more and more independence and the effects of the surgery and anaesthetic diminish, they begin to hope that the time is nearing for going home. This anticipation is usually delayed until the patients feel 'ready' in themselves.

> I understand and accept the need to be here, but it's getting near the end now – at least I hope so. I'm waiting for doctor's rounds so he says, 'Pull the stitches out and you can go home.' At least, they're the words I'm hoping to hear.

Interpreting the Experience[13]

As the reality of the patients' experience of hospital and surgery unfolds, they receive a constant input of information from without and within. The story, which commenced with the surfacing of the problem, is changing and developing.

Individuality is evident in the way stories are recounted. In addition, incompleteness within the story tends to be tolerated. The following account of a conversation between the researcher and one patient illustrates how patients reinterpret information into lay terminology. This man has retained what he perceives to be the information of immediate concern to himself. A meaningful story has been compiled despite obvious gaps in his understanding of the actual surgical procedure. It seems this ignorance is tolerated because the full story is known to the person who 'needs' to know – the surgeon – the expert.

Do you know what is going to happen in your operation?

Vaguely. As far as I know they are going to open it here and they cut part of it out, which part I don't know. I know Mr [   ] did say that they would have to cut away part of the stomach which will make it that much smaller. 'For a period of time you just have to have small meals and more often,' he said. Eventually the stomach will extend itself, possibly not to its full extent, but will reach a stage where I will be able to eat a larger meal. I don't know how long that will take though. I imagine it will take several months.

Interpreting the Experience is a continuing task for patients as they negotiate the passage in partnership with the nurse. The work of analysing incoming information and adding it to the story as known to date, and then synthesising all elements into an integrated whole, proceeds regardless of the efficacy of the incoming information. Information may be wrong, conflicting, or incomplete; the interpretation may be flawed; or the reactions of the patient may be unforeseen. Because nurses are the most consistently present persons, they are significant participants in the information giving. They also have access to the patients' reactions to their interpretation of events as they occur.

During analysis of the data, it became clear that several new elements were appearing in the patient interviews in relation to this construct. As more and more information about themselves in relation to the problem and its amelioration becomes available for use, two subconcepts can be identified: Developing Expertise, and Monitoring Events.

Developing Expertise[14]: From a very early stage in the field work, the notes contained reference to the presence of what was described as 'patient wisdom'. Each new event which involves the patients is added to a growing repertoire of knowledge about themselves in relation to the ongoing passage. As the information is analysed and integrated into the patient's subjective experience, there is an increasing ability to interpret events and take independent action on the basis of the wisdom gained through experience.

I had a really sore stomach so I had a couple of Paracetamol and then about half an hour later I felt really quite sick, as if I was going to be sick . . . . Never had aspirins or Disprins in the house or anything like that so that's why they probably bowled me over. So I think I'll just have one if she brings some back. Two is too much.

I feel funny again now. It's [the urinary catheter] clotted again. I can tell. It hurts like fury.

It's not too bad now. I keep moving around a bit. If I don't sit down on a hard seat too often it'll be alright.

Yesterday it [the dressing] was put there but I don't think it was put on the best way. They sort of just wrapped it around. But this time I put it around properly myself . . . . So, as soon as I did it, it was better straight away.

I'm feeling good now . . . . No clots, not since I've been keeping it [the catheter] pressed every now and then and it's running fairly well now. It's running good.

Despite increasing wisdom about their own situation, patients may feel this is not recognised by the staff and they may submit to an intervention which they do not believe will be successful. One patient had repeated problems with urinary flow through his catheter.

It played up again! Oh, it was terrible! Like nothing on earth! . . . . So they gave me a couple of pills. I said, 'Pills won't do me any good!' So I took them . . . . And that's what it was – the blasted bag! . . . . But, anyway, they put a new bag on. It's been as good as gold since then . . . . I knew the pills wouldn't do any good. I was positive.

Patients may feel confident enough in their understanding of the situation to assist the staff when they feel they have forgotten something.

I think there's been one thing overlooked. I'm supposed to be on a fluid balance – measuring input and output. She just took one away. I hope she measures it because she told me to go to the toilet and give an MSU [mid-stream urine sample] and didn't give me a bottle so she obviously had no intention of measuring it, but she should be. I'll tell her.

This increasing expertise about themselves in relation to the surgery gives patients confidence about future self-care. It can result in a feeling that the time for going home is approaching, even in the presence of a continuing limitation, because patients begin to feel they have the ability to manage alone.

Everything is good and going along, but I am ready to go home now. I won't be silly. I know when I am ready to do a bit more each day with my leg.

The patient gains wisdom in relation to specific issues such as the impact of medication.

The linctus is not bad. It did the job. But I liked the lozenge.

Last night wasn't too bad. I like the valium better than anything else they give you.

At the time of admission patients already possess considerable expertise about themselves. There is a growing wisdom arising from experience about what works and what doesn't.

I like eggs but they tend to constipate me. That is another thing I have to watch. I had milo by mistake for afternoon tea and I was half asleep when I said milo, but I think it constipates me . . . . I'll get my husband to bring up some tangelos. They're the best thing for it.

Sometimes I say to [my husband] at night, 'My back's sore. I feel it's a tense soreness.' I've just got to unwind my back and I like nothing better than a read. So I say, 'I'm going to just have a good old read. I must read for an hour before I go to bed or my back will be dreadful.' And it's only letting the tension go and relaxing – and it does.

Although patients vary in their ability to express this wisdom, there is considerable evidence of its existence. Such expertise, when acknowledged and encouraged by nursing staff, changes the relationship between nurse and patient to one of mutual and complementary expertise.

Monitoring Events[15]: Monitoring, as identified in this situation, has a strong evaluative component. Experience has given the patients a growing expertise associated with increasing confidence to reveal their judgements. Indeed, no part of the patient's experience is immune from comment. The examples of patient evaluation identified in the data were usually subjective and personal.

In the following three excerpts, the patients have reflected on their initiation experience and evaluated it in comparison to their previous hospital experiences.

. . . the nurses, they were very nice too. I am impressed by the friendly atmosphere that is clearly apparent in this ward which wasn't there in Ward [   ] and, in fact, it was a very noisy ward . . . the click clack of all the thousands of heels that clattered up and down the corridor . . . . The occasions when the phone has rung here it has only been a muffled sound – whether it is the bell or it is all the carpet . . . I am impressed by the decor as well. It's a nice modern place.

You see, a lot of them [staff] don't like the old people – and that I *do* know! . . . . I can pick it in the way they talk . . . . I haven't seen it at all today.

Oh well, the whole procedure went quite well, I thought. They're quite attentive and, as I say, I think the nurses have been mucked around by the doctors. I suppose it's the old story in hospitals but I think it shouldn't necessarily be like that. I'm giving you this as a comment – a serious comment. I think there could be a routine that doctors observe as well as others and it would make everybody's job easier.

The behaviour of staff members is evaluated even in personally stressful situations. In the following examples, the patients reflected on the manner of the surgeons who had given them the pathology report after surgery.

And he was direct with me in a nice way. He was very good.

Very matter of fact – 'Good! Fine! Clear! No problems. Appointment in January. See you.'

The patient's evaluation was not always positive as in the following comments from two patients on one doctor.

I had a visit from our lady friend – our lady doctor in here – who tried to explain in detail how Mr [   ] got on in this operation which was no good whatsoever . . . . What she was trying to put across – and she used too many words – was that the operation wasn't successful.

This lady doctor, she was hopeless at putting it in [catheter]. Hopeless! Pricked me inside. I don't think she had much idea about putting it in.

In some comments on the behaviour of individual staff members, patients revealed the criteria they were using in their evaluation.

Some [nurses] are better than others. There are one or two who are not quite as good as the others . . . . I'd say attitude. Some of them have got it and some of them haven't. But when it comes to the point, they're all doing a good job. I think on the whole the standard I would class as 'above average' . . . . Tonight's combination isn't as good as other combinations you get . . . . When things don't appear to be running quite as smoothly, you can sense it. You can pick it up.

The whole procedure went quite well, I thought. They're quite attentive.

As we've gone along, I've been very impressed with him [the surgeon]. He comes in first thing in the morning and you know when to expect him.

Patients were also consistently monitoring their own performance and progress.

I think I've made quite a bit of headway today.

I'm a big disaster today.

And the moment I started eating today and got my tummy settled, I seemed to feel better in myself.

I went down the passage – down there and back. It didn't knock me out.

A better day than I thought I was going to. The same as yesterday wasn't so bad.

The words of nurses are welcomed and evaluated for their significance. Confidence is increased when the patient's interpretation is consistent with that of the nursing staff.

I'm not too bad at all and the kids [nurses] around here reckon I'm doing famous.

Actually, I think Sister seems to be quite pleased with me because she said, 'I think you've been marvellous.' So, she must think everything's gone okay.

Patients actively work their way through a health-related event. In this theoretical interpretation, the patients' work as it is relevant to nursing has been identified. Nursing, through the work of individual nurses, has strategies which can help the patient with this work.

---

[1] This term refers to the patients' work in managing their resources and holding themselves together during the many events associated with the surgical experience. 'Managing' is used in its meaning of 'to be in charge of' (Collins, 1979).

[2] Patients' activity related to restricting their boundaries in order to concentrate on getting through the experience of surgery. 'Centring' is defined as 'focusing' (Collins, 1979).

[3] This term portrays the patients' application of energy, including personal patterns of coping, which they believe will help them to withstand the effects of hospitalisation and surgery. 'Harnessing' is used in its sense of 'controlling so as to employ the energy of'; 'resource' means 'a supply or source of aid or support, something resorted to in time of need' (Collins, 1979).

[4] This phrase describes the efforts made by patients to maintain a state of composure, as least on the outside. 'Equanimity' is used to mean 'calmness of mind or temper; composure; quietude' (Collins, 1979).

[5] This expresses the paradoxical dependence/independence apparent in the behaviour of the patient in relation to 'specialists'. 'Affiliating' is used in its meaning of 'coming into close association with' (Collins, 1979). There is an acknowledged element of subordination in this term which arises from patients' recognition of their need for specialist expertise during a particular experience.

[6] The patient's predominant mode of 'agreement without protest' to the ministrations of specialists whose work is assumed to be beneficial even if it is unpleasant (Collins, 1979).

[7] The words of patients, 'I wanted to fit in with her' were retained and assigned the meaning of 'belonging or conforming after a period of adjustment' (Collins, 1979). The term reflects the patients' willingness to change their normal pattern of behaviour while in hospital.

[8] This term accounts for the independence which patients often demonstrated. 'Autonomy' is defined as the 'freedom to determine one's actions (Collins, 1979).

[9] The pattern of patient behaviour which seemed to have the goal of helping them to get through the experience of surgery. In this context, 'surviving' is defined as 'continuing in existence after adversity'; 'ordeal' is defined as a 'severe or trying experience' (Collins, 1979).

[10] This phrase conveys the patient's need to manage the negative consequences of surgical intervention. 'Enduring' is defined as 'undergoing without yielding'; 'hardship' means 'something that causes suffering or privation' (Collins, 1979).

[11] 'Tolerating' means 'putting up with; being able to bear; treating with forbearance'; 'uncertainty' is used to cover the aspects of the patient's experience which are 'not able to be accurately known or predicted' (Collins, 1979).

[12] 'Hope' was used by patients – 'I hope it's all over' – and 'possessing' means 'owning' (Collins, 1979). The concurrent work of Hinds (1984) in the concept of 'hope' is acknowledged.

[13] This term is a continuation and further development of the concept identified in the Beginning.

[14] This term describes the patients' growing wisdom about themselves and the experience. The reference by Stevens (1979) to the patient's 'expertise' predisposed the researcher to recognise this in the data.

[15] The evaluating behaviour demonstrated by patients is described in this term. 'Monitoring' is used in its meaning of 'observing and recording the activity or performance of self and others'; 'events' refer to 'anything that happens' (Collins, 1979).

6 NEGOTIATING THE NURSING PARTNERSHIP: THE WORK OF THE NURSE

During analysis of the field data it became clear that both the nurse and the patient were actively working to progress the patient through the passage. To emphasise the mutual nature of this relationship, an attempt was made to develop a concept in which a nursing action was directly matched with each area of patient work. However, this approach was found to be forcing the data in a way which did not reflect the complex reality of nursing work. Instead, a complementary pattern of nursing work emerged which is unidirectional in that it focuses on patients working their way through a passage. Within it, each category of work is available, singularly or collectively, to assist patients in each and every aspect of their work during the passage.

The work of the nurse is dynamic and sensitive as nursing responds to the immediacy of the patient situation. Nursing strategies are available to ease the path for patients from their entry – Settling In – to their departure from the Nursing Partnership – Going Home. Thus, negotiating is fundamental to the nurse's work during each of these transition phases.

Nursing's negotiation work within the Nursing Partnership fit five theoretical constructs: Attending, Enabling, Interpreting, Responding, and Anticipating [see Table 10]. Both Attending and Enabling contain a number of subconcepts. Elements of a number of these constructs can be identified within a single nursing episode, and within each nursing act. Thus, nursing actions are multidimensional and complex. However, it is easier to explain each concept separately.

Two hundred and seventy different nursing behaviours were identified in the data – patient interviews, nurse interviews, nursing notes and field notes. Analysis of these, using the processes of the grounded theory approach, led to this conceptualisation of the major work of the nurse.

Although it seeks to explain what was happening in the field, this interpretation was not known to the participants and, there-

TABLE 10: Negotiating the Nursing Partnership: the work of the nurse	
Attending	Being Present
	Ministering
	Listening
	Comforting
Enabling	Coaching
	Conserving
	Extending
	Harmonising
	Encouraging
Interpreting	
Responding	
Anticipating	

fore, was not guiding their actions. Rather, it seeks to give an integrated theoretical shape to the actual work of the nurse as observed in the field.

Nursing behaviours which reflect each concept were clearly evident in the data. Some were effective in terms of helping patients in their passage, while others were not. Both negative and positive examples will be presented in the discussion which follows. Qualitative differences could be seen in the work of each nurse in relation to the concepts and their application within each patient's individual passage. However, the emphasis in this work is on presenting the pattern of nursing's work, and it is recognised that any statement of definitive performance criteria within the Nursing Partnership will require further research.

Attending[1]

As the nurse attends the patient – for seconds, minutes or hours – there is a significant sense in which the nurse is accompanying this person through each phase of the passage. Nursing knowledge and skills are exercised within every nurse-patient encounter. The following example shows how the interrelated thoughts and actions of the registered nurse are specific to the situation at hand.

> She had her dressing taken down and her suture line's a bit red and gaping in a couple of places so we had to dry dress it rather than put some op-site spray over it. She was a wee bit reluctant about actually looking at it. She talked about it and shut her eyes while I was taking the plaster off and then I said, 'If you want to have a look, it's still got a bit of gauze over it.' And so she had a look and then shut her eyes again, and when I did take the gauze off she actually did have a look. And she's worried now that she's going to have to go out and have a bosom on one side and not on the other. So we rang the lady from the Mastectomy Association who's going to come and see her tomorrow or the next day . . . . So I think that today's the first day she's actually really thought about it because, obviously, she realises that it's coming closer to her going home and she's beginning to worry about her appearance and so on.

One nursing action – changing a dressing – has caused the patient to react in a way that the nurse identifies and then acts on. The example illustrates that the quality of nursing is dependent on the ability of each nurse to maintain a vigilant presence, ready to apply nursing knowledge and skills to the patient's immediate situation.

Reflection on this excerpt led to four subconcepts, each of which highlights a significant aspect of the nurse's attending work: Being Present, Ministering, Listening, and Comforting. Within all four there are strong affective, as well as cognitive, elements which reflect the altruistic nature of nursing to give another person specialised help through a particular life event.

Being Present[2]: This concept reflects the fact that nursing is undertaken by individual nurses in the presence of the patient or nursed person. By being present, nurses are able to 'nurse' patients in the immediacy of their situation. Nurses adapt and selectively apply the full range of nursing knowledge to patients' ever-changing circumstances in a way that an unqualified person cannot do.

Table 11 contains examples of nursing activities in which the presence of a registered nurse is significant to the outcome.

To illustrate the value of the nurse's presence, two negative examples and one positive example from the data are presented.

After surgery on the eye, patients were told not to bend over or make any sudden movement. However, a nurse was required to guide the patient through the permitted range of movements when

---

TABLE 11: Sample of activities with an identifiable element of 'being present'

Appraising the current status of the person
Making frequent visits to the patient
Responding to call bell
Giving support during painful procedure
Sitting and talking with person in distress
Giving assurance of nursing presence as needed
Modifying actions in response to patient reactions
Giving encouragement
Assisting patient out of bed for first time

---

the opportunity for bending or sudden movement was encountered for the first time. Such occasions were when the patient was washed, sat up, changed, and recovered personal belongings such as dentures and watches. In this situation the nurse is able to coach the patient and manipulate the environment so that harmful movements are not required. One patient experienced severe pain and considerable bleeding on the surface of his eye after bending over from the bed to look into the cupboard of his bedside locker searching for his dentures. The nurse was not present at the time and recounted the episode to the researcher.

> I reminded him about not overdoing it and no sudden movements or raising pressure after it happened. I think one of the reasons that he did that was because I got his wife to assist him with the post-operative wash seeing she was there. I told him not to over-exert himself and I think he forgot – like he needed my reinforcement when I was giving him the wash . . . . After that incident he was very quiet, lying quietly, and he definitely wouldn't exert himself.

This nurse recognised with hindsight that, although teaching had taken place before the event, her presence was required to nurse the patient through this critical first time. By contrast, in the following example from the same day in the same ward, the nurse's presence allowed her to supervise the safe completion of challenging moments in his experience and to observe his ability to cope.

> Well, he's required routine postoperative care really. What I've done is make him comfortable, given him a postoperative wash and mouthwash and started him on sips of fluids. He seemed to be

coping with those quite well until it came to teatime and we thought he could possibly have a few sandwiches and some soup. Just the motion of sitting him up though made him feel quite nauseated so we sat him down a little and he was complaining of slight pain in his eye so I got him an injection of Maxalon and Pethidine. He's been much happier since then . . . . In the meantime, I made sure, you know, that he was less anxious, by doing things for him like making sure a bottle was on hand and getting his valuables out of the locked cupboard. So he's been fairly routine care really.

The second negative example is recounted because it was the one which confirmed the need for the nurse's presence. The absence of the nurse highlighted the impact of her presence that, in the many other patient situations described in the data, had been taken for granted. An elderly patient who required a stick to walk went down to the bathroom on the third day after surgery complete with dressing and haemovac drainage. She described the episode to the researcher later that day.

I had a shower all on my own. Showered myself. I had to cart this thing [the haemovac drainage]. I did ask the nurse round there. I forgot to ask about it when I went but asked one of the nurses round there and she said, 'You just leave it on the floor.' It dragged on the floor while I showered. I am not quite up on it. I was afraid of slipping when I stepped out. I had only one towel that I had here but they [the other patients] told me I should have thrown that one on the floor and got myself clean ones. They are there. You can help yourself but I never thought to. I'm not used to helping myself. I tried to manage with one towel and I was slipping around a bit. I didn't want to slip on the floor.

The marginal note made by this account stated: 'Need for nursing presence'. From this note came the concept of Being Present and its significance quickly became apparent as a key – indeed the key – aspect of the work of the nurse within the Nursing Partnership.

Ministering[3]: Ministering, as used in this context, is attending to the patient by way of nursing care strategies. It was developed as the second subconcept because it reflects the fact that nursing is thoughtful, sensitive action that demonstrates skill and relevance within the patient's immediate situation.

Table 12 lists a sample of nursing actions from the data in which there is a strong element of ministering.

TABLE 12: Sample of activities with an identifiable
element of 'ministering'

Giving pressure area care
Application of calamine to skin rash
Giving mouthwash
Giving hot drink for sleeplessness
Giving postoperative wash
Giving bed pan
Washing patient and changing bed after
    incontinence
Combing and washing patient's hair
Cleaning dentures
Using fan to reduce body temperature
'Milking' catheter for blood clots
Assisting patient with shower/bath/bed bath
Putting cream on inflamed intravenous site
Removing sutures – anal packing – drain –
    IV needle
Changing intravenous fluids
Dressing wound
Giving medications orally or by injection
Recording temperature, pulse, respiration
Recording blood pressure
Completing preoperative checklist

This list encompasses a range of different nursing acts which
progress the patient through the passage and, as a consequence,
towards an optimal outcome from the surgery.

The concept of ministering can be applied to the planned
performance of skills as well as the incidental activities that are
performed in reponse to the changing needs of the patient. For
example, by being present while a patient is having a shower,
nurses can adapt nursing ministrations to the patient's needs by
thoughtfully and sensitively altering their behaviour throughout
the procedure – standing back, giving assistance, giving advice,
giving encouragement or substituting for the patient.

Ministering may involve the nurse in a pain-inducing activity
which is considered to have a beneficial purpose. For example, one

patient recounted his experience of having packing removed from his rectal wound.

> I was given the injection about 11.30 so it would have been about 12.15 before I went to the bathroom and had my saline bath . . . . Tried to remove it first but that was a bit painful so I hopped in the bath and stayed there for about five minutes and then she came and removed the wadding, or whatever. I think that would be a once-in-a-lifetime experience! . . . I was actually feeling queasy just before. I was in the bath and I'd been left for a few minutes. I felt I was about to faint. I was just on the verge when I was sort of finding things sort of twirling around. I was about to black out so I was moving myself over to one side so I wouldn't fall back into the water. Two nurses came in and got me to lie back and take deep breaths. Then they removed the wadding, then I felt the full experience!

Ministering was apparent in the planning for this event: the administration of analgesia beforehand in anticipation that the removal of the packing would be painful; the decision to let the patient soak in the bath to moisten the dressing; the promptness in returning with assistance; and the spontaneous management of the patient's fainting. In all these areas, the nurse made nursing judgements about the situation which led to actions which ministered to the patient's immediate needs. The removal of the packing from such a wound is often one of the more stressful events a patient has to experience while undergoing surgery. Ministering activities, skilfully and appropriately performed, help the patient through such an experience.

Listening[4]: Because of the nurse's continuous involvement with the patient, part of nursing is to listen as the patient reacts to various situations. It is equally important for the nurse to take heed of the patient's answers to probes for relevant information.

Table 13 lists a sample of nurse activities recorded in the data in which the element of 'listening' is apparent.

Evidence of listening was common in the data. However, it, too, was sometimes identifiable by its omission rather than by its presence. Any data on nursing in action could be expected to contain, as this study did, many examples of imperfect exchanges between nurse and patient. For example, a man with an indwelling urinary catheter shared his feeling of distress during an interview. He was certain that the cause of his pain was a mechanical obstruction to the flow of urine and his experience was made worse by his

---

TABLE 13: Sample of actions with an identifiable
element of 'listening'

Listening to patient concerns
Listening to family member concerns
Encouraging patient to speak of anxiety/fear
Sitting down at patient's bedside to listen
Returning to speak with patient as promised
Establishing eye contact
Moving to side of bed to speak with patient
Being sensitive to patient cues
Stopping activity while listening
Listening when patient's wishes differ from nurse's

---

inability to get his message across to the nurses. In this excerpt, there is evidence of the patient's increasing wisdom about the impact of the surgery on both himself and his body. He believes he knows about what will work and what will not.

> It played up again! Terrific pain like nothing on earth. And my wife came in and I told her and she said, 'Why didn't you tell them?' And I said, 'I told them before' . . . . So she went and saw the Sister. So they gave me a couple of pills. I said, 'This won't do me any good!' So I took them. And they came in later and they said, 'Oh well, we're going to flush your tube out.' And they gave me a new bag. And that's what it was – the blasted bag!

The second example is that of a patient who spoke of his urinary frequency during an interview. When the researcher shared this information with the nurse, the latter was distressed that she had not received this information during her own contact with the patient. It seems the nurse has to work to convince some patients she is ready and able to listen, and has the time to do so.

> He never complains much or says very much. You have to really enquire after him and even then he doesn't tell you everything, as I've just found out.

Evidence of listening is apparent in the following comments selected from the nursing notes of four patients. Each one reveals that the nurse has gained a valuable insight into the patient's situation by listening and this has assisted in nursing decision-making.

Pt anxious about surgery and what degree of pain to expect.

Wound area was very painful when moved and she admits to being very scared of moving.

Feels that the yellow sleeping pills [valium] make him too sleepy during daytime and that the need for them has passed.

Did not want a wash today. Face and hands only.

Comforting[5]: Comforting has been included as a separate concept within Attending to emphasise the capacity nursing has to soothe pain, ease discomfort, bring solace and induce well-being in patients.

Table 14 lists a sample of activities within the data which contain an element of 'comforting'.

TABLE 14: Sample of activities with an identifiable
element of 'comforting'

Placing locker within reach
Adjusting pillows
Giving assurance of progress
Responding to patient requests for information
Giving pain relief
Allaying anxiety about painful events
Holding hand and supporting patient through
    painful procedures
Arranging for wheelchair when patient concerned
    about ability of relative to walk to ward
Listening to patient concerns
Assuring patient of nursing presence
Performing procedures with skill

This concept is well illustrated in the spontaneous responses a nurse is called on to make whenever entering into contact with a patient. The registered nurse brings to each encounter acquired interpersonal and instrumental skills and a body of nursing knowledge which are capable of soothing, easing, allaying and giving comfort within the patient's immediate circumstances.

This comforting work of the nurse is consistent with nursing's traditional role. It is also continually challenging. The nurse may be confronted with a range of situations which require immediate comforting as well as interpretation and action. The comforting role usually has primacy while other actions are planned and implemented.

Table 15 lists a cross-section of patient situations which require comforting work from the nurse.

TABLE 15: Patient situations requiring 'comforting' work
from the nurse

Weeping	Vomiting
Sleeplessness	Nightmare
Agitation	Nausea
Pain – severe	Anniversary of wife's death
Pain – slight	Inflamed intravenous site
Feeling cold	Sore throat
Hiccoughs	Discomfort
Rash	Blocked catheter
Dizziness	Abdominal distension
Fainting	Postoperative shock
Bladder spasm	Stress incontinence
Diarrhoea – in bed	Death of widowed mother's dog
Breathlessness	Diarrhoea – on floor
Back pain	Concern for frail husband
Anger	Confusion through misinformation
Headache	Fear of pathology report
Dry mouth and throat	Leaking of blood from drainage
Profuse sweating	Passing of blood clots in urine

One patient became very agitated on his second day after major abdominal surgery. Pain, noise, light, people moving around, strange bed, regular recordings – all had contributed to his state. The nurse comforted him in a number of ways: discussed it with surgeon and administered medication, washed the patient and made him comfortable, changed his bed to a quieter room, darkened the room, drew the screens around the bed, delayed nursing interventions, and gave the patient encouragement to rest. All were very important to the patient.

> The nurse, she's a lovely person . . . the worst is over. I feel much recovered in comparison to how I felt . . .

In another similar situation, the nurse gave the patient an analgesic, placed a sheepskin in position to ease an aching back, drew the screens and encouraged rest. This nursing work also drew an appreciative response.

Comforting expresses the competence of nurses as they react to a patient situation. It is also apparent in planned nursing activities which could frighten the patient. In the surgical wards in this study, nursing attention to the wound, the drainage or the intravenous infusion clearly required a comforting component.

> [ ] took it [the drain] out *so* gently this morning. I didn't like the thought of it. You'd think it would hurt more, but the biggest hurt was the stitch at the beginning.

Unfortunately, attempts to comfort may not always be successful. For example, one patient had been given the news that his surgery had failed and further problems lay ahead. The nursing staff was genuinely concerned about this outcome and sought to comfort the patient by expressions of sympathy.

> All the nurses trotted around one by one when they got the message and sympathised with me which didn't help much either . . . . They've all been helpful . . . . Their sympathy was quite genuine, I could see that.

The nurse responsible for nursing him during that duty was aware that all had not gone well. Her comments at the interview revealed her reactions to his anxiety and his desire for privacy and the difficulty she was having in knowing how to comfort him.

> I found it quite a challenge because he won't *let* you be the nurse. He likes to set the level of the relationship and lets you know when you're intruding.

Although this nurse was aware that her comforting work had not been successful, this was a rare occurrence. Similarly, nurses seemed to have a limited awareness of the importance of this work when its outcome was beneficial. During this study the researcher sensed that the nursing's comforting work was undervalued by the nurses themselves and yet it was important to the patient.

Nurses often expressed this significant work in phrases like 'reassuring the patient', and 'giving lots of TLC [tender, loving care]'. As used by one nurse, the term 'TLC' conveyed the need for nurses to specifically include tenderness, gentleness, and warmth when working with a patient who was distressed on the day following major surgery.

Enabling[6]

Enabling emerged as a major concept which encompasses the empowering dimensions of nursing's work. By means of activities the nurse assists patients to attain the power, means, opportunity or authority to act within their present circumstances. Five subconcepts have been developed to describe the different aspects of Enabling which could be identified in the data: Coaching, Conserving, Extending, Harmonising, and Encouraging.

Coaching[7]: At first the term 'teaching' was applied to this concept. However, there seemed to be a particular element in the teaching role of the nurse which made the use of the word 'coaching' more appropriate. Coaching can be seen in nursing activities which assist patients to expand their knowledge and improve skills performance within the passage. However, coaching does not stop with tuition. It includes a strong element of ongoing support and guidance from the coach throughout the experience, as happens with the coach of a sports team during a game. Thus, coaching is a moment-by-moment activity as well as a formalised programme of teaching in preparation for an event.

Within the experience of elective surgery, the coaching dimension of nursing is easily identifiable. Table 16 lists a sample of nurse activities drawn from the data which contain an element of 'coaching'.

TABLE 16: Sample of activities with an identifiable component of 'coaching'

Persuading patient to accept analgesia appropriately
Strategies for relaxation and movement
Preoperative teaching
Guidance on ordering diet
Self-administration of eye drops
Discussing breast prosthesis
Arm exercises after mastectomy
Passing urine after removal of catheter
Stopping smoking before surgery
Care of wound while in shower
Adaptation to altered body image
Positioning arm to maintain flow of IV infusion
Increasing mobility after surgery

During interviews, nurses often made reference to their coaching work.

> He's anxious, tense, restless and hasn't been resting enough really in the last few days. And I explained to him today the more he rests the quicker it will absorb and the sooner he'll get home . . . . He's inclined not to listen very well.

> We could actually start teaching him to do it [to put drops in] himself if he wants to . . . . We'll teach him tomorrow.

> I've told him what to expect tomorrow . . . . I told him about the importance not to do too much on the first day. You know – no sudden movement with his head or not to be too active, and that we would be helping him with a sponge in bed.

> Normally we do give people soup and sandwiches, but because he is on a special diet I just gave him the tray with the normal-sized meal and I said, 'Don't be in too much of a hurry to eat it. Just eat a little bit.'

> First of all I made sure she knew what nursing procedures to expect – like when she was given her premed and what it would do to her and where she would be going. Made sure she knew when she could have a shower and just made sure she realised just what sort of things were going to happen . . .

In each of these examples, the nurse was fully involved with the patient in the experience as it unfolded. The coaching was specific to the individual situation and incidental as well as planned. By being present with the patient, and involved in ongoing care, the nurse is able to judge the nature of the coaching that is required to ensure that each person has the knowledge, skill and support that are required in the circumstances.

Conserving[8]: Conserving is used in this model to describe the component in nursing which assists patients to maintain their available resources to the best degree so that they are able to meet the multiple, diverse challenges encountered during a surgical experience. In order to assist the patient to conserve energy the nurse may, for example, encourage the person to rest, do something on their behalf, give assistance, or delay energy sapping activities when resources are low.

Table 17 lists a sample of activities which have an element of 'conserving'.

On one occasion a patient had a bad day during his post-operative recovery. Instead of a reduction in the quantity of naso-gastric aspirate, which was a good indicator of progress, the amount had increased. The medical order for nothing by mouth had been reimposed. As a result, the patient felt very tired and rather low. Previously he had been having a shower with assistance. On this day, the nurse increased her assistance to the patient and supported his staying in bed for hygiene care to conserve his temporarily limited resources.

He's been quite tired today compared with yesterday. I mean he didn't want a shower so I gave him an assist sponge.

TABLE 17: Sample of activities with an identifiable element of 'conserving'

Moving patient with minimal induction of pain
Administering analgesia before painful activity
Inducing rest in presence of fatigue
Giving bed bath instead of shower
Assisting with bath/shower
Assisting patient to sit up
Assisting patient to turn over in bed
Grouping patient care activities
Teaching patient strategies for conserving energy
Encouraging patient to indicate when rest is required
    during activity, for example, walking

In another example, a patient who had renal failure and required haemodialysis had received an excessive intake of intravenous fluid which had affected him. The nursing notes give an indication that his nursing care prior to undergoing haemodialysis was primarily aimed at conserving the patient's strength in order for him to cope with the effects of the additional fluid.

Very tired and rather breathless early in duty and left to rest as much as possible.

Extending[9]: Extending occurs when the nurse uses strategies that enable patients to increase the amount and scope of their activity. Once again, the nurse makes the judgement that patients have the resources to manage increased activity. This judgement is translated into nursing actions which increase the range of self-care activities relative to each person's circumstances. Flexibility and creativity on the part of the nurse are essential qualities; the nurse is 'there' for the patient, reacting to achieve a balance between the person's present status and the performance of self-care.

Table 18 lists a sample of activities from the data which contain an element of 'extending'.

In the recovery of one patient there came a time when the nurse judged that he was ready to increase his activity level. In particular, she decided that the patient could manage a shower with assistance although he was loath to take this step forward.

> And then I've given him a shower which he actually, I think, quite enjoyed. He was a bit reluctant about going.

TABLE 18: Sample of activities with an identifiable element of 'extending'

Withdrawing nursing presence
Reducing assistance to patient
Changing from bed bath to bath or shower
Putting hand bar on bed to facilitate movement
Teaching patient to instill own drops
Administration of pain relief before activity
Transfer of patient into open ward

This extension of his actions was accomplished with the result that the patient felt able to shower himself without assistance the following day.

> Didn't want a hand with his wash or anything.

It is common for nurses to gradually withdraw their assistance so that it becomes necessary for the patient to look after themselves more. Although a nurse may be present with the patient over a number of days during daily hygiene procedures, the nursing role is different each day. This is apparent in the following sequence of nursing notes made on successive days during the post-operative experience of one patient.

> Full sponge given.

> Bathed this morning – enjoyed by patient.

> Up to toilet and bath. Managing well with minimal assistance.

Assisted with shallow bath as necessary.

Supervised with bath. Patient slightly unbalanced [unsteady] at times.

Accompanied to bath but only a little assistance needed with washing back. Managing on own quite well.

On the following day the nurse withdrew so that patient bathed independently and dressed herself ready for discharge.

Harmonising[10]: The fourth aspect of Enabling is to ensure synchrony in the patients' environment and within themselves in relation to the present situation. This requires the nurse to be present with the patient, observing, listening and interpreting, in order to identify any inconsistency. Thereafter, the nurse is able to use methods to help restore harmony. In some cases, nurses may have to act on behalf of the patients, but more often they will work with the patients, giving them specialised assistance as they strive to maintain or attain harmony during each moment of an evolving passage.

Table 19 lists samples from the data of nursing activities which have an element of 'harmonising'.

TABLE 19: Sample of activities with an identifiable element of 'harmonising'

Adjusting pillows
Placing locker within reach
Adjusting bed height
Selecting and arranging pillows and bed linen
    according to surgery and patient condition
Ensuring privacy for rest
Obtaining soft pillow
Placing bell within reach
Providing sheepskin for backpain
Using fan for high temperature
Providing additional bedclothes
Placing urinal/bed pan within reach of patient
Settling patient for night
Positioning patient for meal service
Fitting hand bar to bed
Positioning arm with IV to maintain flow

Several examples from the data are presented to illustrate various patient situations which may require nursing work to restore harmony. Firstly, the patient may be uneasy as a result of conflicting information, as was the case with one patient who had been given two different explanations about the procedure of her upcoming surgery. On the day of surgery, the nurse assigned to her care for the day became aware of some inconsistency leading to confusion on the part of the patient.

> There were two ways they could have done it and I asked Dr [ ] this morning exactly what was happening. He said what he was going to be doing and explained the other way it could have been done, but that wouldn't be necessary for her. Whereas, last night they probably thought it was going to be done the other way in which she would have had the suture line . . . . So she was quite pleased to understand that.

Several patients spoke of being given as many as three quite different indications of how long they could expect to be in hospital. In the following example the disharmony remained unrevealed until she finally asked the surgeon seven days after the surgery.

> [The surgeon] just said they want to watch it to see if I need a skin graft. Then I said to him when did he think I might be going home because I hadn't a clue when I might be going, and he said if everything went alright it could be about the middle of next week . . . . In the clinic I thought Dr [ ] [the registrar] said I would be about a week. About an hour later when I had to get some forms filled in [ ] [a medical student] said, 'Yours is only a small one. You'll be out in a couple of days' . . . . I said to my husband, 'It doesn't seem as if it's going to be too big. Sounds as if it's only going to be a couple of days' . . . . Now I am sort of more settled. I realise now that I will be longer. A couple of days passed long ago.

Harmonising also involves selecting nursing actions which will assist patients to attain consistency between themselves and the physical or social environment. If, for example, patients are restricted in what they can or are permitted to do, the nurse will seek to manipulate the environment so that it is in harmony with this status. In practical terms, the nurse assesses the patient's situation, visualises what the person may need to achieve maximum control, and takes steps to make sure it is available.

> I made sure a bottle [urinal] was on hand.

> And he was quite pleased that he was given a hand bar to pull himself up on. That made his mobilisation much easier.

> She's still using pans by her bed at night, but that's because she can't make it to the toilet in time.

In one situation, the nurse discovered that a patient was not drinking enough fluid. On investigation, the nurse discovered that the patient did not like the fluid supplied and was able to change it to one that he liked. This led to his adherence to the therapeutic regime.

> And he's allowed 30ml of water – which he doesn't like – so we've added a bit of lime to that, and an ice cube – and I think that's pleased him.

Encouraging[11]: Within its repertoire, nursing has a variety of actions which can be used to inspire patients with confidence or courage. Encouraging is particularly required in situations where patients are a little uncertain, afraid or unwilling to extend themselves. It is a component of many nursing actions and is related to, but not the same as, coaching and extending.

Table 20 lists a sample of nurse activities from the data which contain an element of 'encouraging'.

TABLE 20: Sample of activities with an identifiable element of 'encouraging'

Assisting patient to view wound and consider the resulting alteration to body image

Encouraging patient to increase fluid intake

Encouraging patient to breathe deeply

Encouraging patient to speak of anxiety/fear

Allowing patient to make decisions

Encouraging movement in bed after surgery

Encouraging patient to walk for the first time

Inducing hope

Encouraging patient to rest

Giving patient confidence to trust staff

Patients may be afraid that there will be pain or discomfort if they move. In spite of explanations about the importance of movement, the patient may remain still. The nurse may consider that the best form of encouragement is to be present during the specific activity which is causing concern, perhaps holding the patient's hand or otherwise giving guidance and support. In this way, a nurse works to give the patient confidence and to confirm that a particular action is appropriate to the circumstances.

On occasions the nurse's encouraging may be fairly assertive.

> . . . because she's been in a medical ward and she'd had a coronary and she'd had a lot done for her – nursing-wise – she was very demanding at the beginning of the morning. When she came into hospital, she felt we did everything for her. We got the comb out and combed her hair and everything – which I don't mind doing if she needs it but she could do it. So I quietly got over to her that if she could manage, it was better for her to do it. So she did do it in the end. She's quite independent now.

> He also needs to be pushed a bit, I think, because he has a tendency to lie just in one position and not do a single thing for himself.

Nurses often used the word 'encourage' when describing their nursing care. The following examples reflect that the presence of the registered nurse provides specific opportunities to encourage the patient.

> He needs encouragement with fluids. Hasn't been drinking very well lately. His urinary output has been low . . . . He's eating really well. It's just his fluids. You know, you have to keep on going in and offering it to him. Like, before he used to drink without you asking but now you need to encourage him . . . . then all of a sudden he's cut down on his drinking. He had a bit today but that's still with encouragement.

> She's been quite bright – she just needed a bit of encouragement to be out of bed and doing exercises. She seemed to be sticking to her bed quite a lot. And she's a lot better. She only had a couple of drinks – she needs a lot of encouragement with that. Otherwise she's good.

> And he's just feeling a little bit grotty and he needs some positive reinforcement that he's getting better . . . . I've encouraged him with his deep-breathing exercises and coughing because of his chest.

Interpreting[12]

Throughout each episode within a Nursing Partnership, the nurse is continuously interpreting the patient's status, circumstances, requirement for nursing and responses to intervention by all members of the health team. Interpreting has many constituent elements, which include observing, monitoring, analysing, translating, contextualising, synthesising and decision-making. There is an element of interpretation in each nursing action as the nurse adjusts to the patient's presenting situation. The outcome is influenced by the nurse's perception of nursing and what it can offer in a given situation.

Table 21 lists specific examples of nurse behaviours with an element of 'interpreting'.

Examples from the nurse interviews will be used to illustrate different aspects of the interpreting work of the nurse. In the first group, each nurse has reached a conclusion about the status of the patient after observation and interaction.

TABLE 21: Sample of activities with an identifiable element of 'interpreting'

Making decision to consult medical staff
Conserving patient energy
Extension of patient activity level
Modifying nursing care plan
Writing nursing notes
Clarifying medical and other information
Problem identification
Selecting appropriate nursing response
Description of patient and status
Change in orders for nursing care

I think she's had quite a hard time – a lot to cope with – and I think it's a lot to bear at the moment . . . . she sort of needs a lot of TLC or something, I think.

He is a bit apprehensive but he's not very vocal about how he's feeling. He likes to pretend that he's a big and brave man not to complain about pain even though it's obvious from his face that he does have some.

He'll just take it in his stride because he's used to so many things, probably.

His whole attitude was one of wanting to give up because his shoulders were sagged and his head was cupped in his hands and he sat on the edge of the bed in a total attitude of hopelessness.

Interpreting is closely interwoven with other nursing work; there-fore, the nurse's analysis is consistently linked with action. This is illustrated in the following two reflections by nurses on the care of patients during the previous duty.

> Well, physically his condition is really stable. All his observations are stable. He's putting out lots of urine and he looks good. His colour's good. But he's extremely uptight! Very tense. Even though he appears to be quite well covered with his pain relief, when you go to move him or do anything he immediately starts to breathe very quickly and tenses up totally. So he needs a lot of reassurance. He also needs to be pushed a lot, I think, because he has a tendency to lie just in one position and not do a single thing for himself. I think that's basically his problem at the moment.

> Mr [ ] was in quite a bit of pain about 4 o'clock this afternoon both in his penis and, it seemed like, his bladder. I couldn't work out whether or not he was getting bladder spasms but it seemed like he was. So I irrigated his catheter and got quite a few clots back and some very dark haematuria. It didn't seem to help him but his catheter was draining well all along. It hadn't stopped draining. And he had Codis and he seems to have settled down now . . . . When he sits up is when he gets the pain. I don't really know why that is.

The monitoring aspect of Interpreting is most apparent in the nursing notes as specific patterns of reporting on the status of patients is evident. This is particularly so immediately after a patient's return from undergoing surgery, as is illustrated by the following notes from one patient at the end of the morning shift.

> Returned from OT 1130hrs. Obs now 4hrly and stable. Drowsy but rousable. Has not taken any oral fluids as yet and HNPU. *Drugs* – Omnopon 20mg IM 1500hrs for anal discomfort. *Wound* – No ooze. Is packed with 2 green swabs. ? further orders for same.

By the end of the afternoon duty, the progress of the patient was also reflected in the notes.

> Good post-operative afternoon. Obs 4hrly and stable. Tolerating oral fluids and eating small amounts of food. No wound ooze. UTT x1.

The amount of monitored information which is recorded in the nursing documentation is variable, as it depends on the type of surgery and the presence of therapeutic measures such as suction or intravenous infusion, as well as the individual nurse's decision on what to enter in the notes at the end of the nursing duty. In the following example, the night nurse coming on duty has considerable information on the status of the patient during the afternoon.

> *Intake* – IV Barts 12hrly infusing due at 0430hrs. Tolerating fluids and had 150ml soup for tea.
> *Output* – HNPU. Nil ooze from wound. H'vac drained 30ml. No vomiting, nausea or BM.
> *Recordings* – Now 2hrly. P 72-80. BP 170/70 – 190/90 T 36.4 House surgeon aware of BP. Recordings are stable. Could be QQH overnight.
> *General* – O2 discontinued at 1800hrs. Omnopon 15mg and Stemitil 12.5mg IM given at 1730hrs, with good effect. Omnopon 15mg IM given to settle at 2200hrs. Post-op wash given. Moves well when encouraged. Needs reminding to do post-op exercises. Heel protectors in place. Visited by husband twice.

The nursing notes also contained nursing interpretations of abnormal events. Four examples are given to illustrate this. Considerable variation in the format is apparent. Specific reference to the status of the patient during and/or after the event is rarely noted. Neither is it common for nurses to record significant nursing work in the context of the presenting patient situation, for example – situation – nursing action – impact of action.

> Confused and disoriented overnight. Asking for husband and stating why he wasn't there, how he got there, why didn't he stay? Slept for most of night.

> Patient said he had a nightmare and removed his IV cannula. IV replaced by 1st on.

> BP dropped to 72/40 at 1630hrs. Seen by Dr [   ]. IV fluids increased. 1 unit of whole blood over three hours.

> BP dropped to 84/60. House surgeon notified and pt given 1 unit whole blood. Recs ½ hourly while blood in progress – f/satis at present . . . . Appears comfortable.

Another source of information on the outcome of Interpreting is the nursing care plan – in particular, the section where nursing problems are entered. In this study it was consistently apparent that nurses were not entering nursing problems in the care plan despite evidence in the nursing notes and/or interviews. Only three of the 21 patients actually had problems identified after the initial plan was prepared on admission. The seven stated problems were:

Patient 1: 'Pt appears to have little concept of time'
'Potential problem – retention following removal of IDC'
'Deafness'
'Potential problem – ability to manage once discharged'

Patient 2: 'Pain'
'Productive cough'

Patient 3: 'Pain and discomfort'

It is significant to note that the four problems identified in Patient 1 were entered at the time of rewriting the care plan 10 days after surgery. Thus, it became apparent that nurses found it difficult to use problems as the basis for planning individualised nursing care, despite their having been identified.

Responding[13]

Many nursing actions result from a nursing interpretation of a particular patient situation. Such actions may be spontaneous and occur only once, or they may be planned and continued over a period of time. This responding work is not predetermined, although it is consistent with nursing's scope and function. Rather, it is variable according to the nature of the presenting situation and the choices which the nurse perceives are available.

Table 22 contains a list of nurse activities encountered in which there is a recognisable element of selective 'responding'.

Responding is present when a nurse refers a problem for partial or complete resolution by another health professional, usually a member of the medical team.

> And other than that he's been up to the toilet a lot with diarrhoea which he's found a bit disturbing but we got some codeine phosphate charted for him and that's had a good effect.

On several recorded occasions a nurse found herself choosing to respond to a patient's situation in a way which was contrary to that person's wishes. At such times, the nurse tried to persuade the patient to accept the course of action which she judged to be a valid response even though he did not agree.

> He refused pain relief but he appeared quite sore – just from the way he was moving. His movement was quite limited so I gave him pain relief – forced it on him – and he seems a lot better since then.

In this example the nurse's interpretation gave priority to the patient's pain as she perceived it to be. She has noted that the

---

TABLE 22: Sample of activities with an identifiable
element of 'responding'

Bed pan at bedside for patient with diarrhoea
Adjusting pillows for comfort
Providing sheepskin to relieve back pain
Providing privacy for rest during day
Monitoring of blood pressure level when high
Informing medical staff of abnormal observations
    requiring medical response
Emergency measures in response to postoperative
    shock episode
Administration of pain relief
Sitting with distressed patient
Performing procedure in place of enrolled nurse at
    patient request
Modifying care plan following patient appraisal
Administration of aspirin and honey for sore throat
Modification of discharge plan in response to
    patient concern
Administration of laxative for constipation
Irrigation of catheter to clear blood clots
Consultation with medical staff to change
    night sedation
Confirming evidence of progress on part of patient

---

patient's words and her perception of his behaviour do not agree. Her desire for the patient to be comfortable led her to respond in a way which she considered to be in his best interests. A lower priority has been given to maintaining the patient's ability to control his world. This pattern of responding by persuasion was not uncommon in the data.

> She refused pain relief but I made her take a couple of Panadol. I felt she'd actually been a long time without anything and it would be sore.

Occasionally, responding is formalised and recorded in the nursing notes as suggestions or orders for colleagues. The following represent a sample of nursing recorded responses.

Watch heels – protectors on but they need a rub 4 hrly please.

Hospital linctus for troublesome cough.

Pad in situ due to stress incontinence.

Complained of excessive drowsiness this morning. Night sedation recharted.

Complaining of sore throat. Given aspirin and honey for that.

Had 700ml this duty. Water jug taken away. [Patient on fluid restriction]

Anticipating[14]

Anticipating has a predictive quality whereby the nurse visualises the immediate and longer-term futures as they affect the recovery of the patient from a surgical experience, and this is used as the basis for selecting nursing actions which will progress the patient. The visualisation is based on the nurse's increasing understanding of the patient as a person, an assessment of the person's present circumstances, a comparison between the path of progress attained by this patient and others the nurse has had contact with, and some understanding of the potential shape of the future for a person in such a situation. It is linked closely to the nurse's perception of what nursing can offer to make the most of the person's present and future status.

Table 23 lists a sample of nurse activities in which there is an identifiable element of 'anticipating'.

Anticipating is the component in nursing actions which looks ahead. During the preoperative phase, when the patient is new and fulfilment of the purpose for admission lies in the near future, the nurse anticipates the patient's participation in and reaction to the coming experience. This activity forms the basis for decision-making and assumptions about nature of attending and enabling work the nurse will initiate.

> I asked if he was worried about anything just to ask us, but he hasn't asked anything. I just explained to him what I thought he'd want to know. He hasn't really been asking any questions.

Throughout this study, it was apparent that nurses were closely involved in the patient's experience of rest and sleep. In anticipation of the night that lies ahead, nurses ascribed importance to the management of night sedation and the initiation of sleep-inducing activities.

TABLE 23: Sample of activities with an identifiable
element of 'anticipating'

Discussing and demonstrating breast prosthesis
Administration of pain relief before painful
    procedure
Staying with patient in bathroom after injection of
    pain relief
Arranging for visit by voluntary group member
Leaving bed pan or urinal at bedside within reach
Delaying discharge until family support available
Discussing future with patient
Preoperative talk
Withdrawing nursing presence and encouraging
    independence
Guiding patient expectations about upcoming
    events
Placing articles within reach of patient
Writing orders for nursing care

> She had Oxazepam to settle. The girls asked her yesterday about her
> sleeping and she said that she often woke up early in the morning
> and so they got her charted something to sleep in hospital and she
> did sleep well last night.

However, a few days after surgery this patient found herself not
sleeping very well. The charge nurse responded to this situation by
discussing the situation with the patient. This led to a decision to
approach the medical staff for a recharting of night sedation so that
the patient would receive what she was used to when at home.
Thus, there is a constant movement between anticipating and
responding.

> We had a chat about that [not sleeping] and she said that normally at
> home she has valium 2mg which she found suitable. So I've had the
> house surgeon up and she's recharted her valium . . . . So we've
> recharted her valium in the hope that, since that's what she's used
> to, that will suit.

Anticipatory nursing actions often refer to the immediate future. As
nursing is concerned with the moment-by-moment experience of
the patient, the nurse is able to take action in anticipation of a

positive effect during an upcoming event. This was observed in nursing activities such as the administration of analgesia before taking the patient through a painful procedure.

> I gave him some morphine 10mg intramuscularly and then half an hour later bathed him, removed his packing and he's now resting on his bed.

This same patient was waiting with apprehension for his first bowel motion after surgery. As the time approached, the nurse counselled him about what would happen. Her actions reflected her anticipation that the patient would manage the situation better if he knew what to expect: the experience would be painful, it would induce unpleasant sensations, and help would be available.

> And then later on he rang the bell and I ran in and he said his bowels were going to move and I said, 'Well you can just go to the toilet and move your bowels and we'll see. If you feel it's too painful, ring for me, if you need anything.' And I said, 'You're going to feel hot and funny because you do when you have your first bowel motion.' So he went and his bowels moved and he said he felt a bit hot but it wasn't that painful and he was just going to have a bath. So he's quite happy.

The patient confirmed that the anticipatory work had been accurate.

> Knocked me for six when I had the first one this afternoon. Had to lie down. Seemed to settle then.

> Staff Nurse told me she told you that you would be hot and cold.

> Yes. She wasn't far wrong either!

The following excerpt demonstrates that when nurses act they consider present, past and future effects. In this case, the nurse attends to the immediate situation and anticipates his future.

> Actually he's been quite good today. He's had no pain relief at all. He's had an assist sponge and he's been up for a walk by himself . . . . He seems pretty cheerful, you know, and chatty . . . . He's on oral fluids now and they're 30ml an hour which he's tolerating okay. He's burping less than he was a couple of days ago . . . . He's pretty lucky actually because his suture line looks absolutely beautiful – no muckiness or anything. It's lovely. I think once he's rid of his IV and his nasogastric he'll just be up and away really.

Anticipating may be undertaken by the nurse to forestall a negative situation and/or to facilitate a positive state. Inherent in anticipating is a nursing-oriented visualisation of the immediate or longer-term future of the patient.

This discussion has focused on the nurse's work to ease a patient's path. Evidence suggests that the nurse has to focus on the immediacy of the patient's situation to ensure the patient benefits to the full from the application of nursing knowledge and skills. Thus the nurse is continually appraising the patient's status to ensure nursing's work remains relevant.

[1] This multidimensional concept encompasses the nurse's key work of being with the patient during the passage. It conveys the meanings of 'giving care, paying attention, serving, accompanying, devoting one's time, providing for the needs of' (Collins, 1979).

[2] This term arose from a theoretical memo made during substantive coding. The phrase describes nurse's work of spending time with the patient – being there and being with – as the patient negotiates a passage. It came from one of the meanings of attend – 'be present at' (Collins, 1979). The concurrent work of Gardner (1985) and the earlier work of Paterson and Zderad (1976) are acknowledged and served to validate the decision to emphasise this element of nursing work.

[3] The nursing work of actually giving care to meet the needs of a patient. It came from one dictionary definition of attending – 'to give care, minister' (Collins, 1979).

[4] This term is used in the sense of 'taking heed of, paying attention' (Collins, 1979). It stresses the importance of giving patients an opportunity to express themselves, hearing and seeking to attach meaning to what they are saying.

[5] This describes the nurse's work of 'inducing a state of well-being, relieving pain and grief, supporting, soothing, strengthening through bringing ease' (Collins, 1979).

[6] The empowering work of the nurse by which means the patient is helped to make beneficial progress throughout the passage.

[7] This term was derived from its use by Strauss to mean the giving of 'guidance as the patient moves along step by step . . . not merely because he needs to learn skills but also because some very surprising things are happening that need explanation' (Strauss, 1970, p 110). The concurrent use of the term by Benner (1984) is acknowledged.

[8] The nurse's work of 'protecting, preserving, and carefully managing' the patient's resources (Collins, 1979). The use of this term by Levine (1967) 'keeping together' is acknowledged and contributed to the researcher's sensitivity to this work in the data.

[9] This term is used in its sense of 'adding to, enlarging' the scope of the patient's functioning relative to his circumstances (Collins, 1979).

[10] The purpose of the activities undertaken by the nurse to achieve 'accord, consistency, balance, congruity' within the patient and between the patient and the environment (Collins, 1979). The concurrent use of 'harmony' in relation to the status of the patient by Parse, Coyne and Smith (1985) and Watson (1985) is acknowledged.

[11] This term arose from the data itself, 'He needs encouragement.' It denotes the nurse's work of 'inspiring the patient with courage and confidence to take action, stimulating by approval and help' (Collins, 1979).

[12] The nurse's 'translating, explaining the meaning, construing the significance' of aspects of the patient's situation.

[13] The nurse's work of 'reacting' to aspects of the patient's immediate situation (Collins, 1979). It has the added component of being 'favourable' or beneficial to the patient.

[14] The nurse's 'foreseeing and acting in advance of' (Collins, 1979). Actions may intended to 'forestall' the unwanted and/or 'cause [a desired goal] to happen sooner'.

7 LEAVING THE NURSING PARTNERSHIP: GOING HOME

Throughout the Nursing Partnership, the patient and nurse work to negotiate the path of the patient through the passage. Thus, the work of both nurse and patient, as discussed in Chapters 4 and 5, continues until the patient is discharged from hospital. However, there comes a time when the focus moves from the present – being nursed – to the future – without nursing. At this time, the activities of nurse and patient expand to include work which specifically prepares the patient for the transition of leaving the passage and going home.

In this study, the decision to discharge a patient was made by the medical staff. However, this decision could be, and in some instances was, influenced by the actions of both the patient and the nurse. Such actions were primarily initiated by concern for the patient's personal circumstances, that is the non-medical aspects which the patient had revealed to the nursing staff. Despite this opportunity for collaborative decision-making, both nurses and patients tended to acquiesce to the decision of the surgeon, which is usually not confirmed until the actual day of discharge, although a tentative date may have been established earlier in the patient's hospitalisation. There was no evidence of formal discharge planning in nursing work.

Consequently, the terms 'probable' and 'possible' were commonly used by nurses and patients when they spoke of the time of the patient's discharge. This uncertainty is illustrated by the nursing notes and interviews of one patient in the three days prior to discharge.

Three days before discharge:

Notes: For possible discharge at weekend.

Nurse: He'll probably go home at the weekend . . .

Patient: . . . he indicated I could expect to go home probably before the weekend, so I interpreted that as Thursday, but probably Friday.

Two days before discharge:

> Notes: For possible discharge on Friday.

> Nurse: He's probably going home on Friday morning.

> Patient: So I'm not coming home on Friday definitely but it looks pretty likely I will be home Friday.

Day before discharge:

> Notes: Looking forward to possible discharge on Friday.

> Nurse: He's still hopefully going home in the morning.

> Patient: . . . about 4 or 5 o'clock he'll probably wander around and have a look at Mr [   ] and come over to me and I'm expecting him to say, 'Well, yes, you might as well clear off in the morning.' He'll probably have another look in the morning.

Although there was a degree of uncertainty, the indications were clear that both nurse and patient had, at least, a tentative goal at which their efforts could be aimed. Indeed, work before the final confirmation would seem to be essential because patients tended to leave as soon as possible after the decision was made. Haste may be a characteristic component of the transition out of the Nursing Partnership unless nurse and patient attend to their transition work prior to the medical decision.

Going Home: The Work of the Patient

The data indicated that patients work to ready themselves to leave hospital and to resume life at home, and the nurses use specialised knowledge and skills to facilitate this transition. However, from the final interviews with patients after their return home, it became apparent that 'going home' did not mark the patient's return to the pattern of living that existed before the onset of the problem which necessitated the surgery. Rather, it was only a step, albeit a significant one, on the patient's road to recovery from this ordeal. Following discharge, the patients found there was still a lot of work to do and that problems related to the surgery could still arise.

Four concepts which reflect different dimensions of the patient's preparations for going home were generated from the data: Maximising Readiness, Making Arrangements, Discovering Requisites, and Resuming Control. Although they co-exist and interrelate with each other and also with the concurrent activities of negotiation, each will be discussed separately with supportive extracts from the field data.

Maximising Readiness[1]

As discharge became a possibility, the patients' growing expertise in relation to their status was revealed as each would assess the likelihood of the surgeon saying the time for going home was at hand. The patient had usually learned some of the factors which would influence the surgeon's decision.

> Well, if it's clear tomorrow, I wouldn't be surprised if he says I can go home Monday – if it's as clear as it is now.

Often patients would sense the confirmation within themselves that it was time to go. This seemed to come from a feeling within the person as well as from the cues given by others, especially medical and nursing staff.

> Every day I used to look forward to being able to do a bit more, but suddenly I can do it all and there's nothing to look forward to other than going home.

> I wasn't surprised when he said I could go home.

> I think they intend to take the plaster off and have a look and say, 'That's alright. Go home.'

When the patients' sense of readiness seemed to be confirmed by the external cues, even though the final decision was usually not made until the actual day of departure, then the patients were able to prepare themselves to go home to the full. At such times, the resumption of full self-care would be increasingly apparent. However, there were occasions when patients were actually receiving confusing messages which were inconsistent with their own feelings. Such an experience threatened the person's ability to get ready for going home. In the following example, the patient felt ready to go but received no confirming message from the medical staff.

> I don't know what's the story. He just said, 'See you tomorrow,' and walked away. I'm just on holiday now, it seems like.

This patient actually went home the following day.

Despite an awareness that they were ready to go home, patients clearly anticipated that there would be some residual effects from the surgery which they would become aware of as they made the transition from hospital to home.

> Well, I feel remarkably well lying in bed. I guess I won't have so much energy when I'm moving around.

Experience proved to the patients that life does not return to 'normal' for quite a while. During the home visit, patients retrospectively reflected on the impact of the surgery.

> It affected me for a while too. I was surprised, you know. It took the stuffing out of me completely, it did – for a while.

> Just shattered a bit . . . . I'm not feeling the best . . . . I'm starting to come right.

One patient expressed anger as she reflected on how unprepared she was for going home. She felt that specialised assistance should have been available to help her.

> I knew nothing about what I could expect afterwards. I mean, not just in hospital but when I left hospital and went home. I didn't know I would be so tired. I was a bit, resentful isn't the right word, a bit annoyed that I wasn't prepared for going home. I was just dismissed that morning. [The surgeon] came round and said 'Well, you've got your running shoes on. The job's right. Out you go!'

For those patients whose problem had surfaced with a crisis pattern, a degree of uncertainty about the long-term future had to be acknowledged as they prepared themselves to go home. These patients reflected on this during the home interview and revealed that their newly discovered vulnerability had made them less secure.

> . . . you sort of realise that things are – they can't guarantee it won't happen again. Something could happen where it [cancer] comes up somewhere else . . . It doesn't really frighten me. I suppose, having my faith and that, I accept these things more than somebody that hasn't got any. Not that I want to die or anything. I hope I can keep on living for a good while.

> It makes you feel you don't know what's around the corner. I mean, things you took for granted are no longer. I don't feel so secure now . . . . Well, I just think, 'What might happen next?' – all the things that can happen.

This second patient also spoke of the impact of the experience on her husband who had been ill himself in recent months.

> I think he realises I'm not to be taken for granted . . . and I think it's given him the chance to do something for me and I think he likes to do things for me now.

While the presence of a life-threatening problem requires some patients to re-examine their view of life, some patients may also need to ready themselves for an immediate future of uncertainty relating to the outcome of the surgery itself. If no resolution occurs before discharge, a patient has to give due attention to managing this uncertainty when planning to go home. A period of waiting may be necessary before the surgeon can confirm a positive outcome has been achieved.

> He said there's some doubt about the nerve at the back. He can't quite see that. He's not sure whether or not that's been damaged in the past quite unrelated to the cataract . . . . so that's still an unknown but we'll have to wait and see.

> Mr [   ] was also mentioning that there's a bit of soft cornea there that he may have to tighten up the stitches.

> Apparently I am going to have it [frequent diarrhoea] for a couple of months before things settle down.

> The only bit I'm worried about is that I've got quite a bit of fluid [under the wound] . . . . He said the district nurses would watch it and they would get in touch with him, but he said I might have to have a needle – whatever he means – drawn off I suppose.

Thus, in readying themselves to go home, the patients in this study had to incorporate the impact of the experience into their view of themselves and their world, as well as their pattern of daily living. Both immediate and longer-term issues required work from the patient with support from the nurse.

Making Arrangements[2]

All patients spoke of the need to make arrangements for the time of discharge. This means that going home requires specific planning activities on the part of both the patient and others, particularly family members. Usually arrangements had to remain tentative until final confirmation of discharge was received.

> It's only a matter of a phone call . . . .

> So I'll wait until tomorrow and then it's a question of when he thinks I can go home. And then there's a multitude of arrangements to make at home because my wife's got things on which she'll change if necessary to suit the convenience of my discharge . . . . I'll get everything worked out when I've seen him.

> My husband got a surprise when I rang and told him. I have been saying to him to get some shopping in case I came home for the weekend . . . . I will get a friend to take me home or I will get a taxi.

Even obtaining clothes to wear home requires a degree of organisation.

> I've got some clothes here. I'm not going home in pyjamas.

> My wife brought in my clothes last night.

If given the opportunity to name their own time for discharge, patients tended to choose a time which suited the activities of other family members. When the confirmation of discharge was delayed until the afternoon, this seemed to cause more problems for family members than those made in the early morning.

> I could have gone out today but it would have been a bit of a gallop and she had other things on as well so I said I wasn't crashing to go out . . . . So I'm definitely going out tomorrow.

One patient who was expecting to go home became a little upset when the surgeon passed through the ward around midday and, within the patient's hearing, said he would be back later in the afternoon to see his patients.

> If it's go home, then it's a frantic call to the wife to come and get me. I'm a bit annoyed. If he'd come in here first of all – the three of us – and the way he goes through, it wouldn't have taken him five minutes to do the three. It's possible that the three of us are going home. You know, we could have got things organised. Now it's going to be a bit more awkward 'cause she may go shopping after work and things like that. Whereas, if I'd got her at school, she could have come straight in. We've just got to sit here and wait it out.

Although the day of discharge was a medical decision, there was evidence that nurses could negotiate with medical staff and with patients on the arrangements for the patient's departure. Nurses revealed both flexibility and inflexibility in their willingness to fit in with the personal circumstances of the patients in this study. For example, one patient who lived 50 kilometres from the hospital, and whose wife worked near the hospital, planned to go home with her at about 5 pm when she finished work. He was reportedly told by nursing staff that this was not acceptable and his wife had to take leave from her work to pick him up and take him home. By contrast, two patients, one in the same ward as the previous patient, had their discharge delayed when nursing staff recommended to the surgeon that this should occur. In the first instance, the patient unwillingly accepted the decision that he should remain in hospital for an additional day; in the second, the patient initially sought the delay, albeit indirectly, by her expression of concern that no help was on hand.

The first patient, an elderly man who resided in a town some 70 kilometres from the hospital, was planning to travel alone by bus then train and then bus to his home. By the fifth day after surgery he felt ready to go home. However, the charge nurse did not agree and asserted her judgement.

> I said, 'Can I go today?' 'I suppose so,' he said. The Sister said, 'I have got him down for tomorrow. If you have got someone to take you home you can go today.' I haven't got anybody, so a day won't make a lot of difference.

The second patient was an elderly woman whose husband required assistance with his own serious chronic illness, and who lived 60 kilometres from the hospital. On being told she could go home, she became anxious that no help was available that day, although an elderly sister-in-law in another city was available to fly down in a few days. Unfortunately, despite early indications that additional arrangements would be required, discharge planning was not initiated by nursing staff until the medical discharge was confirmed.

> My own doctor is away on holiday I gather, and I had the two other doctors he's usually with. And he just said, 'Go home today and we'll make an appointment for you to come back.' I think he said Thursday or later in the week. But then I said I wasn't really going home today to anybody that could really do anything for me. He said, 'Well, stay here till Thursday,' but then the Sister said, since I've been talking to her, she said, 'Go home Wednesday,' and she'd have help arranged.

This study has clearly revealed that patients do make plans about when to go home, how to get home and how to manage when they get there.

Discovering Requisites[3]

Going home means leaving the ordered environment of the hospital and the specialised services of a variety of personnel. At home, patients have to look after themselves as much as possible. While some help may be available, the person is usually the primary care-giver. Therefore, each person needs to find out what after-care is recommended by hospital personnel – nurses, doctors, physio-therapists, dietitians, and others. However, there is a significant element of chance in discovering this, because the patient often does not know what information is required, from whom it should be sought, and when it is complete.

Several patients denied receiving any guidance on after-care when they were interviewed after their discharge.

> No instructions whatsoever – not from anyone.

But most patients agreed that they had received some specific written or verbal guidance on what they should do to look after themselves at home.

> Just got this stocking and I've got to wash it out each night. She said I would possibly have to wear it for twelve months or so.

> I had a doze-off in the afternoon. I obeyed the instructions – 'Rest up for an hour or two in the afternoon.' That's just what I did.

> The physiotherapist came today and I've got to continue my exercises. She told me I was quite good today so I'm going home with reasonably good arm movements.

> I have to have a bath after every bowel motion. I rang work and told them I'm getting out, but I can't go back to work till next week. He said, 'Yes, it's a bit hard. I can't let you off to go home and have a bath.'

> I've got my diet sheet. It's good. Nothing restrictive about it. There's a lot you can eat. All I can see is the quantities will be the important thing . . . little and often.

Most of the instructions given to patients were primarily aimed at continuing the healing process. However, many of the patients in the study experienced unexpected problems after going home and were less aware that they had been prepared to cope with these. Therefore, when these did occur people often found themselves having to develop their own ways of managing.

The kinds of problems which patients spontaneously shared with the researcher in the final interview at home are listed on Table 24.

TABLE 24: Post-discharge problems reported by patients

Severe headache
Needing to sleep during the day
Inability to sleep
Inability to get comfortable in bed
Giddiness – dizziness – heart 'patter'
Feeling weepy
Feeling 'sick'
Fatigue after activity
Inability to manage a full day's work
Feeling tired 'all the time'
Chest pain
Feeling 'depressed'
Feeling 'nervy'
Pain
Discomfort
Delayed healing of wound
Severe bleeding
Diarrhoea
Loss of sensation in area of wound
Collection of fluid under suture line
Itching
Oedema and ascites
Infected intravenous injection site
Getting dressed after mastectomy
Swollen hand after mastectomy

Most patients seemed to have been given advice on how to manage any pain which they might experience after going home.

> I had to take quite a few Panadol for pain.

Some were offered sedation to use at home.

> They gave me Halcion tablets – 21 of them – when I came out of hospital.

However, most of the problems which did arise were not amenable to pharmacological relief. Guidance on issues such as what kinds of problems might arise, when and who to call for help, and what strategies to use to manage temporary problems was not consistently received by patients.

One kind of knowledge which is required before discharge is the recognition and management of reactions to actually going home. One patient, who had appeared to be apprehensive during much of his hospital experience, described a pattern of behaviour which caused him concern several hours after he returned home.

> I was feeling bad. I eat something and it sort of repeated in me and I start to have wind comes up throat. I feel funny. So we called him . . . . It's because of coming home the doctor said. That what he said. After that I pick up.

In this situation the patient seemed to be experiencing a reaction to leaving the hospital and going home. At least three other patients also revealed a temporary reaction to the transition from hospital to home during the final interview. Two of these patients associated the presence of visitors with the reaction.

> There was a constant stream of people that afternoon and I thought, 'I can't cope, can't cope!'

> During the afternoon we had visitors and I got quite a depressed feeling. I don't know why. Everything seemed to be on top of me yet I was feeling quite well. But I sort of felt that I wished I was back in the security of the hospital ward . . . . Perhaps it was because I wasn't feeling very bright. I was getting quite a lot of aches and pains down underneath the ribs there.

The other patient ascribed her reaction directly to the impact of going home.

> I think you feel as though you are in a different world. That world is going on outside and you're in this one and it takes a little while to adjust when you come out again . . . . You miss it all at first when you first come home.

During the home interview, one patient who had undergone surgery on his prostate gland was quite distressed. He was passing a lot of blood in his urine and this was associated with severe pain. He was greatly concerned. Once again, he did not have access to the knowledge which would enable him to judge whether or not this was 'serious' and what he should do about it. He knew it was most unpleasant and unwelcome.

> I don't know what to do. It's red. It's red blood. You do urine and you have almost stopped and it's very hard to get more. Then you stop and all of a sudden blood comes pouring out. That's what it is. It's blood, straight blood. No doubt about that.

Yet another patient described the onset of a serious problem and demonstrated that she had ascertained what to do in case of real emergency [a haemorrhage] but not before it reached that stage. Initially she felt 'rotten', and this progressed to a major haemorrhage some 10 days later. It signalled a general deterioration in her health which was caused by the progression of the chronic liver disease which had necessitated the surgery. Her husband reacted to the haemorrhage by calling the ambulance, but she had previously instituted her own coping strategies when she became aware of the more generalised indications that all was not well.

> In fact, I think I went home too early. I couldn't cope with anything. I had to get my sister over to stay with me. My husband said he could cope but he was useless. It was so sore. The leg ached and ached. I didn't even want to get up. I made myself go to the toilet and I made myself walk. If I could have just laid there without moving I think I would have. I felt rotten . . . . Just feeling off colour – just feeling as if there's something wrong and you can't pinpoint it . . . . But I wasn't thinking of another bleed to that extent. So, of course, it was rush in and just transfusions until it subsided again.

In preparation for the resumption of full independence when arriving home, patients have to ascertain what they need to do to look after themselves as prescribed for an optimal recovery. Requisites take two forms. Firstly, there may be a need to continue activities commenced in hospital such as exercises, diet, medication, and treatments, and modify these as progress continues. Secondly, there is a need for the person to be given guidance on appropriate actions to take in the event that problems do arise. These requisites are known to the various groups of specialist hospital personnel who have been involved in the patient's care. Some of the problems which did arise were transitory; others signalled problems requiring specialist intervention; a few became real emergencies necessitating an ambulance callout. Patients demonstrated a willingness to learn management strategies when they were made aware of them by the staff member concerned with that aspect of their care, and/or through the agency of the nurse. In particular, they valued an opportunity to sit down with a trusted staff member – a nurse – near to the time for discharge to review the experience and discuss the time that lies ahead as they go home.

> Sister's on tomorrow and she will be able to give me a few ideas as she is very good. She usually makes sure she has a chat, doesn't she?

I think there is a need for a bit of time so you can talk things over.

This great white coat thing . . . you don't get the same responses from nurses. You can ask them more. You feel they are more on your level . . . . You really do need to find someone you can trust to give you the answers if everybody isn't.

Resuming Control[4]

As patients prepare to go home they are also getting ready to assume more control over the way in which the usual activities of daily living are carried out. In addition to taking responsibility for the self-care requirements prescribed by hospital personnel, patients are now required, once again, to make decisions about what they should and should not, will and will not, do. Before going home, patients are already thinking ahead and anticipating an incremental increase in activity as they gradually return to a more usual pattern of daily living.

When I get home I'll just have to take it gently.

I am not going to be a stupid fool and rush around and mow the lawns and that sort of thing. I am going to take it easy for the next few weeks.

During the home interview, patients shared the methods they had used to manage their lives after leaving hospital. They often realised the need to conserve energy as this seemed to be at a premium for many patients, whatever the nature of the surgical intervention.

It's interesting, isn't it – an operation on your eye which is over so quickly and still has its after-effects.

This patient described his first few days after going home and the way in which he coped with the fatigue.

I came home on the Tuesday night. The Wednesday I virtually slept all day and it was not till Thursday after lunch that I started to get up and wander around . . . . I just slept for about a day and a half.

There was also a need for patients to make decisions about the modified routines they would follow, at least initially, until they felt able to fully resume their usual pattern of daily living. During the final interviews, patients revealed that they were making self-management decisions and evaluating outcomes.

The hard part's still getting dressed. For the first nine days I wore the same frock. That was the only one that opened right down the front.

I think this time I went back to work a bit quicker, even on the glide time . . . . I think I thought I was a lot better than I was. The same with the concreting yesterday. This morning I felt quite 'had it' and I was up at half past 6 and ended up going back to bed until about 1 o'clock. I felt I had had it and I knew I had had it.

I got the bright idea of putting about an inch and a half of water in the bath and just sitting in it. The water didn't come up to my groin [wound] and I could wash my back and everything better and soap myself better. I told the district nurse and she said, 'I won't tell if you don't!'

I'm a bit mixed up inside . . . Towards night-time, I'm getting tense . . . . I think I've been subconsciously a little scared of even trying to go to sleep [pain due to insufficient blood supply to leg] . . . . I've had to swap sides in the bed so I can hang my leg over the side.

I have taken my wedding ring off. I thought I would be prepared – like the girl guides – just in case it swelled up. I would be sorry if I hadn't taken it off, but it hasn't swelled up.

In resuming autonomy, the patients were also making decisions on the extent to which they would comply with the recommendations of hospital personnel. Away from the hospital, people make judgements on how long they will continue to comply and the degree to which they will modify the self-care instructions they have been given.

They gave me Halcion sleeping tablets. I took them for 14 days. I'm keeping one or two up my sleeve. I thought I might get a reaction and I thought I didn't want to get in the habit of taking them.

I've still got to be careful. Fruit – you know when I eat fruit – fruit doesn't agree with me. Apples or pears are alright. Green peas is not very good either and even cabbage not very good. To tell you the truth, sometimes I eat too much. But if I eat a little at a time I feel better. That's the way I'm supposed to eat.

Torvan and Mogadon and aspirin – I was taking those and I thought it's one of those that is giving me a headache so I've cut them off the last few nights.

The patient's resumption of autonomy is a major part of going home. This signifies the formal return of decision-making authority back to the patient after the shared pattern which characterises the hospital experience. Self-management means that choices have to be made in the absence of helping people. The work of both patient and nurse within the Nursing Partnership can provide patients with opportunities to prepare for this critical time.

Going Home: The Work of the Nurse

While there was no formal discharge nursing plan in use to guide nurses in their work of helping prepare people for going home, in their documentation and during the interviews nurses did reveal an awareness of progression in the patient's status. Dynamic change and incremental movement towards self-care proved to be generally characteristic of a passage through the experience of surgery. Consequently, nursing time and episodes of contact with the patient tended to reduce as the patient neared the time for going home.

With the final decision about the actual time of the patient's discharge usually being in the control of the medical staff, and delayed until the actual day of discharge, there was a continuing element of uncertainty among nurses about the time available in which to prepare the patient for this transition experience of going home. Despite this, the nurse had available many cues — from the status of the patient, from the behaviour of the medical staff, from previous experience — which gave an indication of when the patient was likely to go home.

I gather he's going on Tuesday. Everything's planned for Tuesday.

I wouldn't be surprised if he goes tomorrow. They don't usually keep them long.

He's going home tomorrow.

He's probably going home at the weekend.

The negotiating work of the nurse precedes and then co-exists with the onset of specific nursing work aimed at preparing for the patient's discharge from hospital. It seems almost inevitable that this work is undertaken in the presence of a degree of uncertainty about the actual time of discharge.

Two separate but interrelated concepts were developed from the data to identify the additional nursing activities that assist the patient's transition out of hospital and out of the Nursing Partnership, Appraising and Supplementing.

Appraising[5]

A major part of the work of the nurse is concerned with assisting the patient to regain the capacity for self-care in the activities of daily living and with selectively giving assistance. This is achieved by constantly appraising the patient's status and deciding what nursing work is required during each episode within the Nursing Partnership. Appraising, as it occurs at the time the patient is preparing to go home, is as significant for the patient as when it happens during Settling In.

Although there was no formalised discharge nursing assessment, the data indicated that nurses were making judgements about the patients' status in relation to their situation as the time for going home drew nearer. Firstly, after progressively increasing the person's ability to look after themselves as fully as possible, the nurse seeks to specify the residual limitations. Secondly, the patient's understanding of the surgery, the after-care, and the future are assessed. Thirdly, the nurse ascertains the nature of the home environment into which the patient will be going in order to match self-care capacity with the home setting – both the physical environment and the available family support. Finally, there is a review of the community resources which could be called on to assist the patient with temporary or longer-term support after discharge.

Most patients in this study were managing their diet, hygiene, activity level, and elimination almost, if not completely, independently by the time they went home.

> He's been up and about – independent with everything. He hasn't required anything.

> The only nursing care she required was having her remaining clips removed. She was completely independent and she was looking forward to going home.

> He's on a soft diet now and really likes that. He was worried that he was constipated . . . so we gave him some PAP. He's just having his antibiotics and that's all the nursing you have to do for him. He's up independently – going to the dayroom and talking with the men in his cubicle. Nothing really to do with the nurses.

One woman who had not been bathing independently prior to the day of discharge was hurriedly given a test that morning. She described the experience during an interview later that day.

> They made me get my own bath. I was a bit surprised that I wasn't going to be pampered and have my bath run for me. I had to run my

own bath and get in and out of my nightdress and bath myself. But I did it! She was getting me ready to go home, that was it. She said, 'If you really want me, press the buzzer.'

Another patient had a large wound in the groin which would require considerably more time to heal and would affect her mobility, her sleeping position and her ability to bathe or shower. At the time of her discharge, this issue had not been fully appraised by nursing staff so that alternative self-care strategies had not been developed to help her as required. During the home interview she described her experience.

> The staff nurse said, 'You can have showers. You should have had one before you left hospital.' And I thought to myself, 'I don't think it looks very good to be having a shower or a bath myself,' And that was the day I was leaving . . . . so I asked Sister and she said, 'Oh yes, you can have one.' Sister came back and she said, 'You haven't had one for two weeks. I wouldn't have one for a bit longer to make sure because you don't want to get an infection in there'. . . . The first couple of nights I couldn't sleep at all. I just lay there with my eyes closed . . . . I couldn't sleep and on and off now I don't sleep . . . . It was always painful to get into bed . . . . It seemed to take ages. Dreadful sort of agony pain to get myself flat. I tried sitting up but I'm not very good at propping myself up to go to sleep.

This study showed that each patient undergoing surgery, no matter how major it has been, will not be totally restored to health and independence at the time of discharge. Indeed, many problems may yet lie ahead of the patient after leaving the hospital and the passage. It is apparent from this study that the nurse can play a major part in easing the patients' transition from hospital to home by appropriately appraising their self-care status prior to departure.

Nurses are also involved in assisting the patient to come to terms with the surgery, its consequences and the nature of the future. Spending time with the patient as the time for going home approaches gives the nurse an insight into the individual's readiness and the additional work both may need to do before the time of departure.

> I explained his drops to him. He understood all the treatment he has to have at home.

> I took her for a shower and she's still a bit iffy about her suture line and what she can and can't do with it. But she does cope with it quite well. She's coming to terms with it really well at the moment.

He's got a little crack there, so when his bowels move it will sting or hurt a bit. We'll have to impress on him that he'll have to keep it [the anal wound] clean and have quite a few baths.

On the day before one patient's discharge a nurse evaluated the effectiveness of a visit from a member of a community self-help group and discovered that important questions remained unanswered.

I think she was a wee bit anxious about it because the lady hadn't really explained where she could get things and what the story was. So, we've got a little stock out the back and we've fixed her up with that and she seems to have that off her mind now . . . . She's tried it [prosthesis and bra] on and she's seen how it looks when she's got something on over the top. She said, 'Oh, it looks even so that's good!' So I think she's all ready to go home tomorrow now.

The nurse working with this patient on the following day revealed that more nursing time, particularly time for appraisal, had been given to the patient during the morning in order to ensure she was as ready as possible within herself for going home.

She was really good today. There's such a big improvement. She said when she went that she's still afraid of cancer but she felt a lot better within herself that she was looking normal and that she was getting back to her own home . . . . I think the cancer bit is really frightening and also the self-image part is really important . . . . She felt good which sort of makes you feel it's worthwhile doing something for somebody, doesn't it. She told me today she feels a fraud because she feels so well . . . . The other lady in the room [same surgery] was very impressed with the fact that she looked so good when she left. So, we've had a good day, really.

Nurses were also aware when things had not gone well and their appraisal indicated their work was incomplete. The uneasiness of one nurse is apparent in this excerpt from an interview just after the patient had departed.

I'm concerned about him going home and I'm not very happy about him at all . . . . He's lost all his 'oomph'. He's a different man from when he first came in. I said to him, 'What are you going to do when you get home?' He said, 'I'll be right as soon as I'm back in my own garden' . . . . I don't know. He's not himself . . . . His whole attitude was one of wanting to give up because his shoulders were sagged and his head was cupped in his hands and he sat on the edge of his bed in a total attitude of hopelessness . . . . So I went and talked it out . . . . I don't know what he's going home to . . . . I don't think his needs have been cared for and whatever is causing his depression, whatever fears he's got, he's not getting support for them.

While this nurse chose not to share this concern with colleagues or attempt to alter the medical decision to send the patient home, two examples were referred to earlier in this chapter where the nursing appraisal had led to nursing intervention. In both cases, the patient's discharge was delayed in order to allow time for the completion of preparations for going home.

A major part of nursing work is to evaluate the assistance and support available from family and friends. While the patients in this study revealed diversity in their social resources at the time of discharge, almost all felt they were able to cope without any outside assistance. One patient lived at home with parents, two lived in flats, three lived alone, and 15 lived in marriage relationships. Six of those who lived with a spouse were themselves elderly and so were their partners. Also, three of the women had 'fragile' husbands whose health status meant they had previously required assistance from their wives. One of the patients who lived alone went home to family members to recover, but two went home alone.

Several patients without adequate family support had already recognised their need and had made short-term arrangements within their family. This information was readily available to contribute to the nursing appraisal.

> Sister said, 'When can your sister-in-law come down?' And I said, 'Well, all the time she's been booked to come tomorrow' . . . . So everything's working out well . . . . She'll cope with helping [   ] [the husband]. That'll keep her busy enough.

> I'm going to my sister's when I get out. I'll stay just a few days until I feel okay to manage on my own.

> Mum's come down and she'll stay till Sunday.

> I have booked my flight home [to parents] for Monday . . . . I'm going to leave him [the husband] to it.

The nurse is able to assist patients by checking that family and/or friends are available to give the kind of assistance that will be required, at least initially, when they go home. In this study, there appeared to be little direct contact between the nurse and the patient's closest helper as a part of a discharge planning appraisal process. Instead, all the patients seemed willing to resume control of, and capable of, managing their own situation and conveying information relating to post-discharge care to their family. However, it seems unlikely that this would be the case with all patients going home from hospital.

Supplementing[6]

Supplementing work by the nurse covers any form of nursing action that helps counter a deficiency of some kind which the nurse identifies in the appraisal of a patient. In this context, the purpose of any supplement is to achieve a broadly defined wholeness in patients and their situations. That is, it may be undertaken to give knowledge, support, and/or assistance that benefits patients as they leave the Nursing Partnership. Such work may be either performed or arranged by the nurse, or both.

As previously discussed, few people in this study actively sought additional support services from the hospital after going home. Most believed they required nothing; a small minority felt that they could not cope alone. However, in each individual situation, the nurse, aware of the range of community assistance available, had the choice of bringing this information to the attention of the patient and guiding the patient's decision-making so that appropriate use could be made of the services.

A significant amount of supplementing work was left until the day of discharge and its performance was dependent on the individual judgement of the charge nurse or the nurse responsible for the patient. The effective use of family support and community services requires the nurse to know what is available and how it could be used to help the patient at home.

In one case, the nursing staff judged that a patient would require additional assistance at home after major surgery. When it was ascertained that he had no one at home and would be alone, he was offered several alternatives, but his constant wish to go home was finally heeded.

He doesn't want to go anywhere but home.

The nursing appraisal was that this patient was incapable of total self-care and his discharge was delayed until a level of help acceptable to both the patient and the staff was arranged.

[The surgeon] suggested that, as I am alone and so forth, I won't get any help at home – which, of course, I haven't had for years and years. He suggested I go out to a convalescent home . . . . I said,

'No, I am not very keen on that. I would prefer to be home.' I'll look after myself even if it kills me . . . . The Sister approached me . . . so, as a compromise with her, I will have meals on wheels.

He also accepted visits from the community health nurse with some reluctance. His preference would have been to have the telephone number of these nurses so that he could call for help if he believed it was required.

I can't see the point of the district nurse coming. She would be pretty busy going the rounds of the various people she is obliged to see and perhaps who aren't as fit as I am, even though I am not too fit at the moment.

Eventually, six patients received visits from nurses in the community health nursing service: two received meals on wheels, two received linen service, one had home help, and two received visits from a voluntary organisation.

He'll go out in the morning and Meals on Wheels will start at lunchtime.

Sister's arranged a bit of home help for her, which I think she was really relieved about.

We rang the Mastectomy Association and they're coming to see her.

The district nurse is going to dress the wound.

One ward seemed to make more use of community support services than the others. The reason for this was unclear, but the attitude and behaviour of the experienced charge nurse seemed to contribute to this outcome. She tried to spend time with each patient on a regular basis and particularly on the day of discharge, and she also actively encouraged her staff to explore the patient's home situation. Whenever supplementary services were initiated, their use was selective and appropriately targetted to revealed needs.

There were often occasions when the patient preparing to go home would have benefited from knowledge that would build up confidence. Nurses often showed they were uncertain about the specific medical plan for the removal of each patient's sutures, clips, and haemovacs, particularly whether or not they would be removed before discharge. Also, if they remained in when the patient went home, who would remove them – staff in the outpatient department, the surgeon or the district nurse? Uncertainty is evident in the following examples from the words of one nurse and several patients.

Nurse: [The wound] gets taken down when she comes back to out-patients, I think. [The wound was actually redressed before discharge and the sutures removed by the district nurse.]

Patient: They didn't say anything about the stitches. I mentioned them to the sister and she said she'd find out. [They were removed the following day before he went home.]

Patient: I don't know whether he said the stitches can come out and you can go home or whether he takes them out or what. [Removed by nurse in outpatient department.]

However, uncertainty was not universally present, as is well illustrated by the consistent references to one patient's sutures over a three-day period. In this case doctor, nurse and patient all knew what was happening.

Day 1: [The surgeon] and Dr [ ] came to see her and had a look at her suture line and told her the sutures could come out on Wednesday.

Day 2: She's having her stitches out tomorrow.

Day 3: I took her sutures out. Good union.

Nurses conduct the day-to-day management of wounds. Therefore, any uncertainty about wound care would seem to be a barrier to the effective nursing preparation of a patient who is getting ready to go home. At the least, the nurse should be aware of the parameters for decision-making and be able to discuss these with the patient.

Although, in this study, the problem was resolved by the point of departure, it often remained an unknown for nurse and patient until that time. Then, the nurse made the arrangements, having ascertained any special preferences the surgeon may have for after-care. Private patients tended to go back to the surgeon in his rooms, while some received an appointment for the outpatient clinic and had sutures removed there. Nurses from the community health nursing service were also enlisted to continue wound management and they gave other supplementary nursing care as required.

The district nurses are marvellous really. It was one long stitch and she said, 'I'm afraid I'm going to hurt you a little bit.' So I just thought, 'Okay,' and I didn't feel a thing! . . . . They popped in once or twice just to see how I was.

As discharge approached, patients often failed to hear, or understand, communications from the medical staff concerning their discharge. At such times, these patients needed additional assist-ance from the nursing staff – explanation, confirmation, listening to concerns.

> I heard the doctors say to [   ], 'Make an appointment for so and so and so and so,' and I didn't gather who or when but she's had her orders so I suppose I'll be told tomorrow.

> This morning he had a little fumble around and he said – I don't know whether he said the stitches can come out and you can go home or whether I see him on Wednesday in outpatient's or what.

Valuable support could be given to patients by providing them with specific guidance on the appropriate helping resource to contact in the event of any problem arising after discharge.

> And if he has any problems, he just rings up.

> . . . the district nurses will keep an eye on it [the wound] and contact him [the surgeon] if there are any problems.

The final entry in the nursing notes tended to summarise both the nursing and medical follow-up information given to the patient by the nurse. Nurses were performing a range of activities which maximised the patient's readiness for going home. Two examples from these entries serve to illustrate this part of nursing's work.

> Discharged home to wife. Follow-up at 2 weeks. Private appoint-ment with Mr [   ] on [   ]. Referral to district nurse. Nursing instruction given. Cont on increased fluids during day. Cut back after 3pm. Explanation of district nurse's visit. To notify hospital of any change of condition – bleeding. Prescription given for soluble aspirin.

> Seen by surgeon. Discharged home this PM in care of wife at 1830hours. Private patient – to make own follow-up appointment in 2 weeks' time. For discharge on Gutt Chloroptic 1% BD and Gutt Maxitrol 1 drop QID. Eye care instruction sheet given to patient. No script or health services required on discharge.

It is evident from this study that the nurse is in an important position to initiate a range of supplementary assistance for patients before and after discharge when nursing judgement suggests they are needed. The purpose of such actions is to ease the person out of the Nursing Partnership as safely and comfortably as possible, secure in the knowledge that the individual's needs have been identified and targetted help has been given. This supplemental work is undertaken in negotiation with the patient and/or the family and is consistent with nursing's scope of practice as portrayed in this theoretical framework.

The final phase of the Nursing Partnership – Going Home – requires both the patient and nurse to undertake their own pattern of work. This is essential to ease the patient's transition from hospital and the supportive work of the nurse within the Nursing Partnership to home.

[1] This term describes the patient's preparation of self for going home. 'Maximising' means 'make as much as possible'; 'readiness' means 'preparation for action' (Collins, 1979).

[2] This term was derived from the data. One patient spoke of his need to 'make a multitude of arrangements' before he could go home, while other patients conveyed this same idea in other words.

[3] This encompasses the patients' need to know what they had to do for themselves at home in order to continue the path to recovery. 'Discovering' is used in its sense of 'determining, finding out, learning, ascertaining'; 'requisites' are those 'essentials, necessities' which patients must undertake to optimise their continued recovery (Collins, 1979).

[4] The patient's activities related to resuming responsibility for self. 'Resuming' is used in its sense of 'taking back'; 'control' means 'the power to direct or determine' (Collins, 1979).

[5] This describes the evaluative nursing work undertaken as the patient moves towards the point of going home. 'Appraising' is defined as 'assessing' the distinguishing characteristics of the patient and the situation which are judged to be significant at this time (Collins, 1979).

[6] This word describes the nursing work of organising supportive community services for patients on their return home. 'Supplementing' is used to mean 'adding to, making up for a deficiency' (Collins, 1979).

8 CONTEXTUAL DETERMINANTS WITHIN THE NURSING PARTNERSHIP

Nurse and patient meet in the complex setting of the hospital where a multitude of factors are operating. These include such diverse elements as the architectural design of the ward, the financial, physical and staffing resources available, current medical practices, the social and cultural support for surgical intervention, and the provision of support services within and without the health-care system to assist the patient. Against this background the nursing service is organised. Staffing patterns, conditions of service for nurses, practice philosophies are all influenced by the social and cultural environment for nursing. In turn, these factors influence the shape of the Nursing Partnership.

As this concept of the Nursing Partnership evolved, it became apparent that there were three specific determinants within the nursing setting which were consistently affecting both patient and nurse throughout their partnership. Thus, they were having an impact on the shape of the patient's passage. Indeed, it became evident that these factors are an essential element within this framework if the model is to closely reflect the reality perceived in the data.

Contextual Determinants within the Nursing Partnership[1]

A hospital ward comprises a group of people collected together because of their need for nursing; this need is caused by the presence of a health problem which usually requires specialised medical intervention. Nursing care is organised 24 hours a day, seven days a week by a group of nurses who have specified conditions of service. In addition, the social sanction given to nursing means that patients enter hospital with some expectation of what being nursed will mean. The service is valued and there is a tendency to think well of its practitioners. Each of these factors influences the relationship between nurse and patient.

As data analysis progressed, the large number of factors that seemed to be influencing the partnership was reduced to three: Episodic Continuity, Anonymous Intimacy, and Mutual Benevolence. These will be discussed with supportive excerpts from the research data.

Episodic Continuity[2]

Entry into the Nursing Partnership means that the patient is in a situation where nursing is constantly available. However, that does not mean that each person is constantly in the presence of nurses. Analysis of the data has revealed that the contact between nurse and patient throughout the passage is episodic. In effect, nursing is seen to be a series of comings and goings as nurses come to the patient to perform specific tasks many times in the course of a nursing duty. Paradoxically, the cumulative effect of the episodes of nursing, spread as they are over the 24 hours of the day, is that patients perceive the nursing as being continuous.

> There's a whole lot of people been coming in and asking me if I was alright . . .
>
> . . . girls in and out all the time.
>
> The nursing care is good. It's still fragmented but − it's someone different popping in all the time and doing different things. But they seem to have everything under control and they're very nice. You know, got a good manner with the patients. They're trained to be good.

As the fieldwork progressed, the short duration and intermittent nature of nursing contact became evident. In order to examine this phenomenon further, a period of constant observation of two patients was undertaken over a nursing shift. Neither patients nor nurses were aware of the observation at the time. Coincidentally, both patients were on their second day after similar major surgery and each was being nursed by a different nurse. They were in two open cubicles within the same room and could be observed, except when the screens were drawn around the bed, from a vacant cubicle in the room. At the time they were the only patients in the four-bedded room.

During the period of observation, one patient received 11, and the other 12 nursing visits, mostly from the nurse assigned to their care. The total nursing time was 53 minutes for one and 63 minutes for the other. Field notes revealed almost identical patterns of nursing contact. Table 25 contains the field notes made on one patient. This clearly demonstrates the episodic, task-focused nature of the association between nurse and patient.

TABLE 25: Observed nursing contact with one patient

0810–0850: Bed bath, change of night attire, mouth care, checking IV, care of nasogastric tube, out of bed for first time, walk around bed, patient sitting in chair, bed made, patient taken for short walk, then assisted back to bed, positioned and nurse leaves.

0954–1001: Nurse enters, aspirates nasogastric tube and records amount, takes temperature, pulse and respiration, places call bell within reach, checks intravenous infusion, checks with patient that he is alright.

1014–1015: Student nurse enters and stands at end of bed, they greet each other with a smile, she asks how he is feeling, responds to his reply and moves to other patient.

1053–1057: Nurse enters, smiles at patient, checks IV, speaks quietly to patient, assists him to move up the bed and leaves.

1106–1108: Charge nurse enters room, stands between patients' beds and greets them one by one, smiling at each and leaves.

1128: Nurse enters, checks IV, smiles at patient and leaves.

1159: Nurse enters, checks IV, fills glass with water and leaves it by patient, records it on fluid balance chart, asks patient if he is alright, he says yes and she leaves for lunch break.

1259–1300: Nurse enters, checks IV, patient has eyes closed, nurse leaves.

1312: Nurse enters with daughter who has gone to get her, tells patient she will get him an injection, he nods and she leaves.

1317–1319: Nurse returns, pulls screens, administers injection, repositions patient, records temperature, pulse and respiration, fills his glass with water, pulls back screens and leaves.

1415–1419: Nurse enters, checks with patient that he is alright, checks intravenous infusion, aspirates nasogastric tube, checks fluid balance chart, refills glass with water and leaves.

In discussion with this patient's nurse at the conclusion of her duty, she expressed surprise that the cumulative total of nursing time was only 63 minutes. She felt she had spent considerably more time with the patient. Analysis of her comments in the interview indicated that, despite the episodic nature and short duration of nursing time given to the patient, the nurse perceived her contact as being continuous. This experienced nurse was only working two days a week in the ward and this was the first day she had been assigned to this patient.

> Right – first of all he seemed bright. Very eager to please, I felt. I gave him a full sponge. Sat him out in a chair, probably getting on for an hour all told. And then I took him for a walk from cubicle four to cubicle two and back again. But then, once he got back into bed he seemed to get progressively more miserable – and his daughters have since confirmed it. And I think it's just because he had a sleepless night and he's feeling a little bit grotty. He needs some positive reinforcement that he's getting better. And – apart from the bed bath, he's on four-hourly recordings – TPR and BP – and they're not bad except at 1400 hours the temperature was 37.9. But he had complained earlier of being cold and I had bundled him up in a cuddly – so whether that helped to bring it up. He's on nasogastric asps every four hours and I got a lot – 130 and 250ml. But he's on free fluids which he's not tolerating. He's tolerating them but he's not drinking a lot – 30 to 100ml an hour. And he's on free drainage of his nasogastric tube but that's drained nothing freely. I've had to aspirate it. His wound's dry. I've encouraged him with his deep breathing exercises and coughing because of his chest. And that's about him, I think. I can't think of anything else. He had Omnopon 20mg and Maxalon 10 at 1320 hours and he had his last dose prior to that at 0630. He had been sleeping so I didn't see any reason to give it to him sooner but he was ready for it when I gave it.

During this period of observation, the episodic contact was almost exclusively with the nurse actually assigned to nurse the patient. The presence of two empty beds in the cubicle meant that fewer nursing visits were made to the room in the course of the duty, but this cannot be assumed to have significantly affected the total nursing time for each patient. Neither nurse gave any time to the other patient while she was in the room.

If this pattern of nursing time and episodes, even including the longer period usually required for morning hygiene care, was repeated over the three nursing shifts in a 24-hour period, each patient would have contact with a minimum of three separate nurses over up to 30 visits, which would amount to no more than three hours of actual nursing time. The cumulative total of nursing contact observed in this instance occurred at a time when both patients required regular nursing attention to the intravenous infusion, nasogastric drainage, pain relief, hygiene and mobility, oral fluids, and recordings of blood pressure, temperature, pulse and respiration.

Nursing episodes consistently became less frequent and of shorter duration as the patients progressively assumed more self-care. This is apparent in the following comments by nurses.

> What have I done for her today? She's been fairly independent all day again. She's had a sponge – just needed her backwash done . . . . Up and about. She's fine. She's had no pain relief or anything really.

> He's just having his antibiotics and that's all the nursing you have to do for him.

> He's been independent . . . . He looked after himself. He showered himself and got up and cleaned his teeth and – yes – he's independent . . . . He hasn't needed any nursing at all. He's just had his diarrhoea and coughing but he's coped with that.

> Well, she's independent with everything. We only made her bed . . .

Episodic nurse-patient contact is understandable when the work demands on the nurse are considered. Regardless of the organisational pattern operating in the nursing team, each nurse seems to be constantly on the move – circulating between assigned patients, the service areas of the ward and the nursing office. During duty, the nurse is expected to be continually available to patients at all time by means of the patient's call system as well as periodic visits. Thus, paradoxically, each nurse has a perception of continuity in the nursing care of each person.

The following three examples illustrate the way in which nurses weave together their episodic contacts with the patient – both planned and spontaneous incidents – into a story that reflects their perception of a continuing nursing presence during the duty.

> He slept soundly. Never saw him awake all night. Well, he had valium 10mg orally to settle. So he did very well. Got him up reluctantly for a shower this morning but he's fine. He's first on the list so he's all ready to go. He's just had his premed and he's ready to go down at 0800 hours.

He got up for a while before tea and he sat in his chair. And I went in after tea, about 1815 hours I think. He'd just got up on his bed and he seemed to be a little bit distressed and upset. He just sort of shed a few tears. I think things were getting on top of him a bit so I talked to him for a while. He was a bit sore and uncomfortable and fed up. I helped him put some xylocaine jelly around his catheter site and he cheered up. He was okay after that. I think he's just wound up. He's very pleasant and cheerful, but sometimes I think it might just be a bit of a brave front. But Dr [ ] came in this evening and told him he could have his catheter out tomorrow so he's quite rapt about that.

Mr [ ] started the day off very badly. When I arrived he was sitting on a pan with diarrhoea and he had been there for some time I suspect. And his drip was leaking back and his pyjamas were soaking, his bed was soaking – absolute misery! So I took the drip out and gave him a choice of a shower or a bath, and he decided on the shower but half way through the shower he decided that it might have been a mistake. It was a bit late by then so we completed the shower. Back to bed and he had his dressing done. He had pain relief and he had quite a long snooze after that. He was a bit agitated for some of the time but not too badly. But he's on valium 5mg tds and that's really helping now. He's still nil by mouth. He's got an IV with vitamins every eight hours. Generally his output was low this morning because of his reduced input. I don't think there's anything to worry about . . . it wasn't until 1400 hours when he'd had a sleep that he said, 'Thank you for how you cleaned up the mess this morning', and then he said, 'Like a veteran!'

This first contextual determinant on the Nursing Partnership is seen as a paradox because, although nurse-patient contact is in reality a series of purposeful episodes usually of short duration, both nurse and patient have the impression of a continuous nursing presence. Against this background, the nurse and patient work their way through the passage.

Anonymous Intimacy[3]

Another paradox becomes evident when attention moves to the nature of the relationship between nurse and patient. From a very early stage in the fieldwork it became clear that patients were having some difficulty in distinguishing between nurses and attaching a name to a particular nurse. The concept of 'anonymity' began to appear regularly in the coding. Even when recounting particular incidents, the patient rarely identified the nurse by name. This is not to say that the nurse would not have been distinguished from others by sight if not by name.

During interviews, when the nurse was guided to speak about a named patient, only on four occasions did nurses begin to describe another patient until corrected. So, nurses were able to link a name with the right patient at the end of the duty. However, it was apparent in later discussions that the majority of patient names were not retained by nurses for long after the nurse-patient contact had concluded. Questions such as: 'Now which one was he?' or 'Was he the [operation]?' indicated that personalising details were not retained after patients left hospital and their place was taken by another, and another. Despite this mutual anonymity, the activities within the nurse-patient partnership are intimate and personal.

In a surgical ward, there is a constant turnover as patients come and go. Nurses are confronted with changes among the patient group almost every day they are at work. In addition to the constant changes in the patient group, the nursing group itself is also constantly changing. The nursing team functions on a rotation of three eight-hour shifts with two days off each week for full-time staff. Part-time staff, who may work reduced hours and/or as few as two days each week, are usually included in the nursing team.

Whatever the system of nursing care, the maximum number of eight-hour periods in which a patient can associate with one full-time nurse is five out of 21 each week. Even if a nurse is assigned to the same patient every day while on duty, the total nursing time may be no more than one hour per duty at the most, and this may occur only on the morning duty, and only when a patient is requiring the most nursing.

Table 26 summarises the number of changes in nursing personnel experienced by each patient in the study. It clearly illustrates the difficulty of providing continuity of patient contact with one nurse in a system which is based on the division of nursing personnel into eight-hour shifts and a 40-hour week.

The assigned nurse may not be the only one in regular contact with the patient in each duty. For example, in three of the wards, students were assigned patients under the supervision of a registered nurse. When a nurse tutor was also present, the patient had regular contact with three nurses during that particular duty. In all wards, specific tasks were centralised to some degree, so that patients tended to have services such as drug administration undertaken by nurses other than the one assigned to them. Finally, there were incidental episodes between the patient and other nurses in the course of a duty. Therefore, it was possible for a patient to be nursed by a number of nurses during a duty.

TABLE 26: Frequency of nursing personnel changes per patient during hospital stay

Patient (in Order of Time in Hospital)	8-hour Duties	Nurses	Duties per Nurse		Maximum Contact With One Nurse (percentage)
			Range*	Average Per Stay	
1	64	21	1–9*	3.0	14
2	49	23	1–5	2.1	10
3	46	21	1–8*	2.2	17
4	36	21	1–6	1.7	17
5	34	16	1–5*	2.1	15
6	33	9	1–6	3.7	18
7	28	16	1–5*	1.8	18
8	28	8	1–7*	3.5	25
9	25	18	1–3*	1.4	12
10	24	10	1–6	2.4	25
11	22	14	1–3*	1.6	14
12	20	10	1–5*	2.0	24
13	19	10	1–4*	1.9	21
14	19	8	1–5*	2.4	26
15	18	8	1–5*	2.3	28
16	16	8	1–5	2.0	31
17	13	7	1–3*	1.4	23
18	10	5	1–3*	2.0	30
19	10	6	1–3	1.7	30
20	10	5	1–3*	2.0	30
21	10	8	1–2	1.3	20

* For the range of number of assigned duties per nurse, the maximum includes more than half night duties when only one or two nurses are responsible for the whole ward

[Which nurse is looking after you?] A variety of them.

There still seems to be a lot of people coming and going – a lot of different people . . . . An uncounted number of nurses!

Analysis of patient interviews revealed that it was exceptional for an individual nurse to be recalled by name. No patients consistently named all nurses who were involved in their care. Even the fact that the interviews took place at the end of a nursing duty did not mean that patients could name those who had cared for them during the duty. According to Table 26, the 21 patients in this study had a cumulative total of 252 nurses assigned for at least one duty. Of these, only 16 nurses were ever specifically named by patients while discussing their care with the researcher.

Five nurses were consistently referred to by name by a total of six patients. The three male nurses in the study, distributed among three wards, were always referred to by their first names. Four patients received nursing from one of these male nurses. As the female colleagues of these male nurses were not named by the same patients, it can be assumed that, because there are fewer male nurses, they stand out from their female colleagues and their names are remembered. A particular female third-year student was also regularly named by two patients. In consultation with the charge nurse, she chose one of the patients in the study for her own case study, and so was assigned to nurse her and a second study patient in the next bed for five consecutive duties – an unusual event. One staff nurse who worked with the third-year student in caring for these same two patients, and continued to nurse them after the student changed to night duty, was also named by both women. While quality of performance was not associated particularly with the male nurses, it was definitely linked with the student and, to a lesser extent, the staff nurse.

The retrospective comments on this student nurse by these two patients made her stand out as no other nurse did.

> That little one [ ], she was only a little thing but she seemed as though . . . like, when she was taking tubes out and things, she seemed gentle but firm. She knew exactly what, and you had confidence in her. You knew she was going to do her best not to hurt you, whereas some of them just take things out and don't sort of help you.

> It was that [ ], she's a gem of a nurse. We all liked [ ].

Ten other nurses and one charge nurse were named on either one or two occasions during a patient interview, but the use of their names was not consistent. Seven were referred to only by their first names. In the remaining three, which included the charge nurse, only the surname was used.

Instead of being referred to by name, specific nurses were occasionally identified by the use of such distinguishing terms as:

'the Dutch one', 'the dark one', 'the one in blue', 'not this one, the other one', 'the one that calls you Lovey', and 'the girl with ginger hair'. It was common for nurses to be referred to using the more impersonal forms 'Nurse' or 'the nurse' or 'she'.

> Nurse helped me. It was very nice. Some young nurse helped me shower.

> I am making water all the time. She has taken one pan away. I thought perhaps I had a catheter in me and I asked Nurse. She said no, it was draining.

> Nurse has just shaved me ready for the morning.

> Nurse helped me out and I sat in the chair while she changed the bed.

> The nurse came in and told us what the operation entailed.

Another common term used when discussing nursing care was the impersonal plural – 'they' – even when referring to the actions of a single nurse.

> Then they came and got me into my theatre things.

> They gave me a pain injection so that made me feel a bit dozy.

> After they put the dressing on, it was very uncomfortable so once they [wife and children] left I asked one of the nurses if they could get to take it [the eye pad] off . . . . I asked if they would and they did.

> They took that [IV] out . . . and they pumped the bladder out.

It seemed that patients were identifying with nursing and nurses rather than individual nurses, in most instances.

> The company's very nice and these frequent changes of female company are a great life. They come and they go and I don't really recognise them next time round because I haven't really seen them very well first time round.

> Later on, when I went for a walk down the corridor I saw Dr [   ]. I said hello to him and told him and the nurse that I had taken these things out but the trouble was, I was talking to the wrong nurse. She didn't know what I was talking about. When I look at a person I don't look at the card or whatever they have got on. They are either white uniforms or green or whatever and it doesn't worry me who is there as long as the person who is meant to be looking after us is there.

I couldn't tell you their names . . . . they were all very good . . . .
No, I couldn't say any special ones at all. They were all exactly the
same to me.

Despite the overwhelming lack of individualisation of nurses by
patients, and the brevity of the relationship with each nurse, the
content of the contact between them was immediately intimate for
the patient – such as being washed, having an enema, using a
bedpan, verbalising concerns, and so forth. In each nursing episode,
patients shed privacy and expose themselves to the ministrations of
a stranger. This submission, unacceptable in other situations, is
possible because such activities are considered to be within the
domain of nursing practice. However, it was obvious throughout
the fieldwork that the work of the nurse is constantly under
scrutiny, and the patient's initial openness to all nurses could alter
in the light of subsequent events.

> One day one old lady that was in there, she wanted one of the nurses
> and I said, Don't get out of bed. Ring your bell.' When the nurse
> came she said, 'The lady over there told me to ring my bell.' She
> turned round and gave me such a look. I thought, 'Next time I mind
> my own business.'

> I couldn't stand it any longer and I called the night nurse. She is a bit
> of an old grump. She does speak but she hardly looks at you. You
> don't know whether you should call her or not.

> Well, there were some people you would ask if you needed
> something and there were other people who you wouldn't . . . .
> You didn't really want to be a bother to anybody and some people
> made it feel, seem, that it was a bit of a bother.

Although there was a lack of individualisation of nurses, patients
were able to distinguish between groups of nurses. On several
occasions, one charge nurse was referred to by name, but the
uniform colour or positional category was most consistently used –
'Sister', 'the one in blue', 'the one in charge'. At the time of the
fieldwork, there were a few remaining hospital-based students who
were commonly identified as 'the one in white' or 'the [ ] year
nurse'. Students from the local technical institute were were usually
labelled as 'the polytechs'.

Patients were able to distinguish between students and registered nurses and seemed willing to be nursed by students. On his
first postoperative day after surgery for repair of an inguinal hernia,
one patient had managed to go down to the bathroom to wash and

groom himself for the day. Some time later he found out that he was to be cared for by a first-year 'polytech'. He refrained from informing the student that he had already cared for himself and submitted to a full bed bath and assistance to get out of bed!

> Well, they have to learn. They don't do you any harm.

Later he allowed each of the group of students to take his blood pressure.

> Well, this morning they were all having a go. They were trying so hard and absolutely hopeless, some of them . . . and you see the keenness in them, you know. Have a look at them in five years' time!

Another patient who had been in the hospital on a number of occasions and who had the opportunity during her present hospitalisation to observe the recovery of a number of patients as well as herself, shared her perception of the difference between students and qualified staff. She observed that, in the beginning, nursing students have not developed skill in inducing confidence in patients. In the following excerpt from an interview, she recounts her own and another patient's responses to receiving nursing from a first-year student who was unsupervised during the performance of a procedure at a critical time for the patient after surgery.

> Some of them are the first-year ones. I don't think you are quite as confident, especially if they are going to get you out of bed when it is your first time out of bed. You feel as if they might hurt you. They don't really know how to hold you as well as one that's in her third year or a staff nurse. They know exactly how to hold you, whereas they are not sure of themselves or of you either. I was trying to do things to help myself. I was saying, 'No, I'll do this and that.' Like the other lady – she was a nervous wreck at even the thought of anything. But she was terribly upset when the first-year one took her down for her first bath after her operation. She was in such a state when she came back. She said she was so afraid she got down on her knees but she wouldn't get down in the bath. I think it was just because it was a first-year nurse.

In addition to inducing confidence in the competent performance of skills, staff nurses were attributed with the possession of more nursing knowledge than students.

> I think they have a bit more know-all, don't they?

At least in the surgical setting, there seem to be few opportunities for closeness of the kind associated with a friendship or an ongoing helping relationship. The 24-hour nature of nursing and the staffing patterns which have been devised to maintain that service mean that continuity exists between the patient and nursing, rather than a single nurse. However, even when confronted by a series of nurses who, as people, are strangers, patients are willing to reveal much of themselves as they receive a variety of intimate services which nursing has the social sanction to provide.

This second paradox, in conjunction with the first, means that the nurse's episodes of contact – for seconds or minutes – with people who are essentially strangers, provide the context within which the nurse performs the work of nursing in partnership with the patient.

Mutual Benevolence[4]

A third and final concept emerged from the data to form a trilogy of contextual determinants, each impacting on the other. It became apparent that the partnership between nurse and patient is one of mutual goodwill. Throughout the field experience, both nurses and patients appeared to be genuinely concerned for the welfare of the other. For the nurse, this concern can be considered as an integral part of the professional role, and is manifested as a generalised inclination to help associated with an ability to translate that disposition into a specialised form of beneficial action.

During interviews the nurses made frequent optimistic statements about patients. Such comments tended to suggest that 'all is well', or soon will be.

> He's really good . . . . I've been really impressed with him today.
>
> I think once he's rid of his IV and his nasogastric, he'll just be up and away really. But he's been doing really well today.
>
> He's doing very well. He's really good. I mean, he had a hernia repair as well, and a laparotomy, so he's done very well, really.
>
> He's good. He's fine, yeah. His eye could still improve a bit, but I think he's quite happy with what's happening to him at the moment.
>
> Well, for a start, when we came on he was a bit tearful and full of pain – a bit wet around the eyes and not very happy about his regression . . . . but progressively over the PM duty he's cheered up and he's back to his normal, happy self.

It seemed that nurses were also trying hard to coordinate their personal and professional perspectives and to avoid expressing negative feelings about their patients. The few personal comments recorded during interviews with nurses tend to be gently positive.

> He's a nice old gent.

> Poor man, I feel sorry for him.

> Oh, he's lovely – he's a lovely man – very pleasant.

> He's really nice. All the dialysis patients are really nice – usually. When you're working in Ward [ ], they're all so nice.

> I found her a very nice girl.

> . . . he's a very pleasant guy, actually. He'll be quite nice to nurse.

> He's fine. He's gorgeous.

When nurses did express personal reservations about, or even dislike of a patient, the reaction was limited and linked to an attempt to understand that person's situation.

> Oh, Mr [ ] – the most aggressive, rude little man – and demanding – that I have ever come across. I have not very often come across somebody so rude. But underneath it, he's quite a scaredy-baby . . . he's a very angry gentleman, that one. And I thought he was just getting rid of some of the bitterness in him at me . . . . So we had a nice little chat after that remark was made and we talked a bit . . . . He feels more relaxed now – getting away from those ugly thoughts.

> . . . but, however, I don't like the man for all that. He's far from easy. But, really, he's quite good as far as we're concerned.

> I find him a very strange gentleman. I think his deafness has a lot to do with the answers you get from him which are sometimes inappropriate . . . . Very amiable kind of man.

In the field data, activities which are considered unpleasant, such as cleaning up body discharges, were undertaken by nurses without any verbal expressions of personal distaste, and negative reactions were concealed from the patient. In the following example, it had been necessary for the nurses to 'clean up' the bathroom floor after a patient had a large loose bowel motion on it.

> At about 1400 hours, though, she had diarrhoea – didn't make the bathroom in time. It was positive to occult blood. And she's a bit miserable following that.

The benevolence demonstrated by patients is genuine and consistent. It is commonly expressed in conjunction with discussion about the personal ministrations of the nurse, especially at times when the patient is unable to undertake self-care. A real warmth was evident in the voices of patients as they shared their appreciation of the nursing staff – collectively or individually – in their own fashion.

> But the attention I've been getting is very good. Quite meticulous! Nice girls.

> The girls are marvellous – they are. They're one hundred percent. I told them. I did.

> I make it as pleasant as I can for them and they make it as pleasant as they can for me.

> Oh, I've had tremendous support from family and friends and I really think the staff here have been marvellous.

Occasionally, when patients spoke of a negative experience which involved a nurse or nurses, there was a tendency to emphasise that the incident did not detract from the positive feelings about nurses as a group.

> Every time, it [pain] went straight away as soon as they flushed it [the catheter] . . . . Well, I asked them to do it before – to give me a flush – to flush out my kidneys again, you see. They said, 'Oh no, it'll be alright.' But I'm not saying much because they're all marvellous – the girls are. Honest, they're all wonderful.

> These young people asking you to relax. It's just absolutely impossible. You are trying your best. It's like trying to drag a bull by it's tail. You can't do a darned thing until the pain has lessened. I was a little brassed off about that but, even so, they are good girls doing a wonderful job, I must admit.

Indeed, the goodwill a patient feels towards the nursing staff, together with appreciation for the assistance given when needed, may hold the person back from expressing negative reactions directly to the nurse concerned.

> And, of course, getting uptight with the nurse. I didn't say anything to her. I would never do that. But it was probably the way I felt, you know. She hurt me a little bit when she put something in here [intravenous infusion] and little tiddly things. It was probably me being upset. But I didn't say anything to her. I just went along with it.

> Not bad really, except when I got an orange cordial drink – this was pathetic – instead of a lemon drink and it upset me because the nurse

wouldn't take my order. It's weird. Just little things. One out of a thousand times when I wanted something and I got what I wanted. The service has been fantastic . . . . That was the only thing – only thing!

Some patients considered the possibility of a small gift as an expression of appreciation to the nursing staff. One elderly man made little mats and distributed these to some of the nursing staff and one house surgeon, as well as to the researcher. Chocolates and orchids were other gifts given to the nursing staff. One elderly woman spoke of wanting to express her appreciation with a gift but was unable to translate the thought into action.

I wouldn't mind shouting the girls but don't know how to go about it, so I'll leave it. They are too busy . . . . If I can manage to do anything for the girls before I go, I would.

The concept of Mutual Benevolence emerged from the data to signify the reciprocal goodwill between nurse and patient. The motivation to nurse, and the internalisation of the humanitarian philosophy inherent in nursing, provide the nurse with the inclination to want to help and the ability to take action. A predisposition on the part of patients to think well of nursing staff seems to be related to the nature of work that nurses undertake. Appreciation was evident in patient interviews, especially when the patient required the kind of activities which others in the community would find it difficult to perform, such as assistance with body cleanliness and care of body discharges. This tendency to mutual benevolence, closely related to the nature of nursing's work, makes it easier for nurse and patient to relate together in the episodes which characterise the Nursing Partnership.

[1] This term was developed to describe the group of emergent factors within the nursing environment which exert a significant influence on the shape of the passage. 'Contextual' is used to refer to 'circumstances that are relevant to an event'; 'determinants' are 'factors that affect' the context in which the Nursing Partnership occurs (Collins, 1979).

[2] 'Episodic' is used to mean a series of 'incidents, events'; 'continuity' means 'occurring without interruption or as a whole' (Collins, 1979). The concept is paradoxical and reflects the shared perception of wholeness in spite of the reality of intermittency of contact between nurse and patient.

[3] The word 'anonymous' was initially used in margin notes and was retained for the concept. 'Anonymous' is used in its sense of 'lacking individual characteristics'; 'intimacy' indicates 'closeness incorporating warmth and understanding' (Collins, 1979).

[4] This term was developed to reflect the goodwill discovered in the data. 'Mutual' conveys the meaning of 'common to or shared by both'; 'benevolence' means actions and feelings of 'goodwill, kindness or friendliness' (Collins, 1979).

9 FURTHER DEVELOPMENT OF THE NURSING PARTNERSHIP

The theory of the Nursing Partnership is in the process of development. Since its origin in the narrow context of a person's experience of hospitalisation for planned surgery, a number of changes have occurred. These have both broadened the application of the model and made it more complete.

According to the literature of the grounded theory method, the emerging theory has value if nurses react by indicating it 'makes sense, by making theoretical sense of common sense' or say, 'That's it, that's just the way it is!' (Glaser, 1978, p 14; Stern, Allen and Moxley, 1984, p 376). In response to a written or verbal presentation on the Nursing Partnership, nurse peers have made the comments such as the following:

It just makes sense.

It's what I've been waiting for.

It feels right.

The model is perfect for the surgical setting; we want to use it.

It has wide application beyond the surgical setting.

It's psychiatric nursing.

It's midwifery.

I'd love to use it.

Concern at what was perceived to be a hospital focus, led more than one colleague to pose the challenge:

Could it be changed so we could use it in the community?

Yet others asked:

Is it only applicable when people are sick?

These positive reactions instilled confidence. Continued reflection and invaluable discussion with colleagues, together with the experience of using the model in a three-year nursing curriculum, have led to some significant changes.

One early change was the decision to use the term 'client' throughout the model. The recipient of nursing in the original model of the Nursing Partnership was termed the 'patient' because that was the term used by all concerned in the field. However, over recent years there has been a move, particularly by those working in the community, to replace 'patient' with 'client'. The argument in support of this move has three fundamental points. Firstly, 'patient' has a close association with illness, and nursing does not only work with the ill; secondly, 'patient' is closely linked to the medical model; thirdly, 'patient' is often considered to imply passivity whereas 'client' suggests more control through its meaning of 'a person who seeks the advice of a professional man or woman' (Collins, 1979).

The term 'client' is used throughout the remainder of this book. Nurses using the model in practice are encouraged to use the most appropriate term for the setting in which they are practising. A 'client' of nursing may be an individual person, family, group or total community. 'Patient' is commonly used when a person has a specific health problem and/or the person is receiving nursing in association with medical care in a hospital or medical centre. 'Resident' may be used in reference to the clients of some long-term agencies.

The revised model will be presented as a whole, with modifications in the definitions of established concepts and an explanation and definition of each new concept. The following headings will be used: The Revised Model, The Beginning, Entering the Nursing Partnership, Negotiating the Nursing Partnership, Leaving the Nursing Partnership, and The Contextual Determinants.

The Revised Model

The revised model is presented in diagrammatic form in Table 27.

The Beginning

Initially, the Beginning represented only the patient/client's experience with a health-related problem from initial awareness to the point of entry into a Nursing Partnership which is associated with its resolution. Now it reflects the work of both patient/client

TABLE 27: The Nursing Partnership (Revised)

The Work of the Client

Surfacing the Problem	Becoming a Client	Managing Self: Centring on Self, Harnessing Resources, Maintaining Equanimity	Maximising Readiness
Preparing for Intervention	Suspending Social Roles	Affiliating with Experts: Acquiescing to Expertise, Fitting In, Retaining Autonomy	Making Arrangements
Interpreting the Experience	Revealing Self	Surviving the Ordeal: Enduring Hardship, Tolerating Uncertainty, Possessing Hope	Discovering Requisites
		Interpreting the Experience: Monitoring Events, Developing Expertise	Resuming Control

The Work of the Nurse

The Beginning	Entering	Negotiating the Partnership	Leaving
Maintaining Readiness	Admitting	Attending: Being Present, Ministering, Listening, Comforting	Appraising
Self	Appraising	Enabling: Coaching, Conserving, Extending, Harmonising, Encouraging	Supplementing
Nursing Protocols		Interpreting, Responding, Anticipating	
Associate Protocols			
Organisational Protocols			

Contextual Determinants

Within the Community
Culture: Materials, Practices, Beliefs and Values
Health Care System

Within the Client
Causal
Environmental

Within the Partnership
Episodic Continuity
Anonymous Intimacy
Mutual Benevolence

Within the Nurse
Nursing Knowledge
Nursing Wisdom
Regulation of Nursing
Conditions of Service

and nurse prior to the commencement of the Nursing Partnership. It is a time of adaptation to a changed situation and preparation for an upcoming experience. The duration of this Beginning phase may be anything from days, perhaps even hours, to years.

The revised Beginning phase is summarised in Table 28.

TABLE 28: The Beginning

The Work of the Client
Surfacing the Problem
Preparing for Intervention
Interpreting the Experience

The Work of the Nurse
Maximising Readiness
Self
Nursing Protocols
Associate Protocols
Organisational Protocols

The Work of the Client

Three theoretical constructs were developed from the field data to identify the work of the patient/client during this initial experience which would be relevant to nursing: Surfacing the Problem, Preparing for Intervention, and Interpreting the Experience.

Surfacing the Problem

This is the process in which the patient/client acknowledges the existence of a problem, adapts to the presence of the problem, makes a decision to seek assistance, undergoes diagnosis and testing, receives information from a health expert on the specific nature of the problem, and, finally, accepts the recommendation that specialist intervention is required.

If the word 'problem' is defined as 'any health-related experience that is, or will become, difficult for a person or group to deal with without nursing and/or other assistance', then the term can refer to anything from the experience of dying, to a health problem such as chronic illness, to a traumatic event, to any experience of surgery, to the experience of pregnancy and childbirth, or to a knowledge deficit.

Nursing is traditionally associated with nurturing people as they pass through the extremities of life – being born, suffering for any reason and dying. People moving through these passages of life remain the primary focus of nursing's work. During a recent television programme a prominent musician, when recounting his personal experience, clearly articulated nursing's privileged role of sustaining people when hope seems gone. He said something like: 'When your guts have been torn out and there's nothing left, you need nursing'. When a person is dying or when illness or disability is present, nursing does have something very precious and meaningful to offer to the person and family.

In the research which generated the Nursing Partnership, nurses were involved in the care of people through a short period of hospitalisation for surgery – a common passage which many, if not most, people have in their lifetime. However, nursing is also a significant partner for people as they pass through positive life experiences such as pregnancy and childbirth as well as the promotion and maintenance of health. In all these circumstances, the nature of nursing's work remains the same, although its expression within a particular Nursing Partnership will vary according to the person's passage and the nursing support required to make progress.

Four different patterns for the way in which a problem may surface were identifed in the data. These remain relevant at this stage in the development of the model, although further work will be required to encompass Nursing Partnerships in which the major focus of nursing's work is health-enhancement and support through positive life experiences.

Evolution – the gradual development of a problem to the stage where intervention by a person or group with specialised knowledge and skills is recommended to alleviate its impact;

Crisis on Evolution – the development of a long-standing problem to a critical state which is now potentially life-threatening and urgent intervention has become necessary;

Anticipated Crisis on Evolution – the evolution of a problem to a stage where urgent intervention is required to reduce the risk of either sudden death or fear-inducing debility; and

Crisis – the sudden presentation of a proven or possible malignancy or other health-related event associated with pain, suffering and death, or a dramatic change in life-style which requires urgent intervention.

Preparing for Intervention

The client takes steps to get ready to enter the Nursing Partnership, and other passages within partnerships involving other health personnel, particularly medicine. The client strives to become equipped with the resources needed to withstand the consequences of the problem and the impending intervention.

Interpreting the Experience

Throughout the experience, a client analyses events as they occur and synthesises them into a meaningful whole. From this whole, details are selected to form a personalised account of events.

The Work of the Nurse

It soon became apparent that there was something missing in the prelude phase of the Nursing Partnership – namely, the nurse's preparation for the encounter. Of particular concern was the way in which standardised protocols which would be applicable in particular settings could be integrated with the model. Ultimately, a multidimensional construct was developed to reflect the requirement for each nurse to maintain a readiness to act – as a nurse, as a nurse in a specific setting, as a partner in health care, and as an employee.

Maintaining Readiness refers to the work nurses undertake to be fully prepared for the initiation of each Nursing Partnership. This includes acquiring the appropriate knowledge, skills and attitudes which are essential to practise safely and to exercise professional responsibility and accountability.

Four distinct areas within this preparatory work can be identified: Self, Nursing Protocols, Associate Protocols, Organisational Protocols.

Self: Readiness of the self includes the acquisition and upkeep of the persona associated with being a nurse. While there is considerable international comparability in the meaning of nursing, each society ultimately stamps its own shape on the role so that it is congruent with the beliefs, values and practices currently in vogue within that community.

The basic nursing programme is a period of socialisation through which each nurse attains the attributes a particular society requires of its qualified nursing workforce at the time of registration. In New Zealand today, the legal requirement that a nurse be safe to practise at the time of registration now includes a specific expectation that the beginning nurse be culturally safe. This development recognises that professional competence is multifaceted and requires the nurse to perform safely in the socio-cultural context in which nursing is given and received. In the years of practice which follow registration, all practising nurses have an obligation to keep their knowledge, skills and attitudes up-to-date. However, dramatic changes in health care and nursing knowledge mean that safe, competent practice cannot be assumed from nurses returning to practice after a period away, or even from those currently practising who fail to attend continuing education programmes or read professional journals. Nor can it be expected from nurses who are newly arrived in a particular society and whose professional socialisation and experience have taken place in another cultural milieu.

In addition, all nurses need to be settled in their own selves, as distinct from their role as nurse. This means that nurses enter a Nursing Partnership totally ready to focus on the person/client rather than on their own personal worries and concerns, and have adequate resources to act.

Pearson's recent comment is helpful.

> The nurse who knows herself/himself can also like and trust the patient enough to work *with* him professionally, rather than *for* him. In this way the nurse recognises that the power to heal lies in the *patient* and not in the nurse. She/he takes satisfaction and pride in the ability to help the patient use this source of power to grow and develop, and become comfortable working with members of other professions (Pearson, 1988, p 141).

Nursing Protocols: Nursing Protocols are the conventions within nursing practice which reflect current nursing theory and experience, supported by nursing research. These form the foundation for the work of the individual nurse within a Nursing Partnership. All nurses have to familiarise themselves with enough of nursing's current body of knowledge to exercise full professional responsibility for safe, competent nursing judgement and practice in a given setting.

Tanner confirms that quality nursing decision-making is associated with the selective application of established nursing protocols to the care of a particular person, '. . . even when the clinician makes conscious use of research-based theories and techniques, he or she is dependent on tacit recognitions, judgments and skillful performances' (Tanner, 1988, p 205). She goes on to link judgement with application of theories to particular situations, 'There are no formal strategies of clinical judgment that can be described free of the context in which the action occurs' (ibid, p 212).

Associate Protocols: It has been common practice for nurses, seeking to define the scope of nursing practice, to classify nursing functions as being either dependent/delegated or independent. Lists of the former are often more numerous, more specific and seemingly regarded as more 'important' – even more 'interesting' – than the nurturative activities which support the person through a health-related experience. In a discussion which highlights the tendency for nurses to practise routine care which adheres to dominant medical and management models, Pearson suggests that patients see nurses as being 'obsessed with the performance of tasks associated with physical care and the support of medical regimes and that they do not fulfil expectations as the humanisers of the health care system' (Pearson, 1988, p 3). This tendency, by nurses as well as others, to give pre-eminence to the routinised performance of delegated tasks denies the reality that when nurses perform a 'dependent' or 'delegated' function they imbue that task with their professional frame of reference.

In this context, the task has undergone a significant change from the original, usually medical, skill. For example, if a medical colleague asks a nurse to remove the packing from a wound following surgery, the nurse will use independent judgement to set the nursing context for the removal – appropriate timing, planning to fit with other client experiences, preparation of client for the event, performance of the task with skill and sensitivity to the person and the state of the wound, and the after-care.

From one perspective, the nurse is 'merely' doing what she or he has been told. This, of course, devalues nursing by prolonging the myth that the purpose of nursing is to 'serve' the client by serving the medical profession. The alternative view, as proposed by the theoretical framework of the Nursing Partnership, is that the nurse offers a specialised service within a team of experts. By working with the client within the Nursing Partnership, nursing facilitates the work of medical and other partners within the health team.

If 'associate' is defined as 'partner, colleague, ally', then associate protocols are those conventions within the practice of medicine or health which nursing can incorporate in the Nursing Partnership. Each nurse can be expected to be thoroughly familiar with relevant associate protocols and the related nursing protocols which transform them into a nursing framework. With this knowledge available, the nurse is ready to exercise full professional responsibility for the safe, competent performance of such protocols, and for the nursing judgement required to blend them appropriately into a specific passage.

Organisational Protocols: Organisational protocols are management conventions designed to bring order to the day-to-day operation of a group, association or institution. Such protocols may be developed by way of a variety of management philosophies, and by different combinations of personnel within the management team. For example, the organisation may be the health-care system at the level of national government, an area health board, a large city public hospital, a private surgical hospital, a small rural maternity unit, a rest home, a community health centre, a domiciliary nursing service, a group of nurses in private practice, a multidisciplinary team within a health agency, or a nursing unit in a larger agency.

In the reality of nursing practice in any setting, a nurse is likely to be required to attend to a variety of types and levels of organisational protocols. For example, a nurse in a nursing unit within a hospital needs to be familiar with such conventions as admitting a client, care of valuables, documentation, collection of specimens, visiting hours, laundry service, meal service, availability and use of equipment and materials, quality assurance, and staffing of nursing units.

As with associate protocols, when organisational conventions impinge directly on the work of client and nurse within the Nursing Partnership, they are performed within a nursing framework. Thus, a knowledge of the nursing context for the performance of organisational protocols is also essential for the nurse.

Entering the Nursing Partnership

In its original form, the phase called Settling In was named from the data. Nurses consistently used this term to refer to the transition phase when the person was admitted to hospital. As used, it seemed to be referring to an ideal outcome following the shared work of client and nurse.

However, because of the association of this term with entry into hospital, it is of limited value and is capable of being misunderstood in a generalised framework applicable in any nursing setting. The focus of the phase is on entry into the Nursing Partnership in any setting. Thus the term 'Entering' is appropriate. Such a straightforward term does not detract from the model because the focus of the mutual work of client and nurse remains clear.

Entering is the transition experience in which the patient/client comes into contact with nursing. Both client and nurse have their own pattern of work to perform during this phase. This work is summarised in Table 29.

TABLE 29: Entering the Nursing Partnership

The Work of the Patient/Client
Becoming a Patient/Client
Suspending Social Roles
Revealing Self

The Work of the Nurse
Admitting
Appraising

The Work of the Client

On entering into a Nursing Partnership, which is often associated with entry into a health agency, the client has a range of work to perform. Through this work, the client, supported by the work of the nurse, accomplishes the concurrent tasks of becoming a client to the agency, to the medical staff and other health groups, as well as becoming a partner within the Nursing Partnership.

Three separate but interrelated patterns were developed from the data to explain the work of the client upon settling in: Becoming a Client, Suspending Social Roles, and Revealing Self.

Becoming a Client

The person must transfer into the client role. This process is assisted by learning experiences at the time of entry, the person's previous experience(s) of being a client, and the facilitating work of the nurse.

Suspending Social Roles

Whether a person moves from home to a hospital or other health agency, or remains in the normal environment, a patient/client reduces activity within, or lays aside, the usual range of social roles and responsibilities for the period of a health-related event.

Revealing Self

On entry to a Nursing Partnership and related partnerships, the new client is required to become exposed, in word and body, to others, especially nurses and medical staff, and to accede to intrusive procedures performed by people who are virtual strangers.

The Work of the Nurse

The nurse has two major tasks to perform during the entry phase: Admitting and Appraising.

Admitting

This theorised nursing work has proved a stumbling block for some nurses working in the community.

But we don't admit people.

However, the term 'admit' has a dictionary meaning as follows: 'accept, allow to enter, give access, initiate, introduce, let in, receive, take in' (Collins, 1979). Given this definition, 'admitting' seems an appropriate descriptive name for this work, but a broader definition is required.

The nurse acts as associate by undertaking a set of tasks on behalf of others – hospital administration, medical staff and other health personnel – to accomplish the patient's admission to hospital. This may well be the case in any nursing setting but there will be considerable variation in what the nurse chooses or is requested to perform. Although these are delegated functions, they are given a nursing perspective and have become an integral part of the work of the nurse.

If there are no such protocols in a particular nursing partnership, then this aspect of the model is not applicable.

Appraising

Specific activities are initiated by the nurse to establish an information base about the particular clients' circumstances which will be relevant to the client's nursing and will guide decision-making during the partnership. In this initial appraisal the nurse will gather and analyse information on the client's prelude experience, the status of Entering work, and the the status of Negotiating work. In addition, guided by the nature of the setting, the nurse will seek to build up a relevant picture of the client's status in relation to other concurrent passages.

The nurse will seek to answer this question: 'What do I need to know to initiate this nursing partnership?'

Negotiating the Nursing Partnership

The major work of nurse-client negotiation through the Nursing Partnership commences at the time of entry and continues until the client leaves the passage. It co-exists with, and supports, the work associated with Entering and Leaving.

Collaboration is required to help the client proceed through the passage as effectively as possible. It is a dramatic moment-by-moment process as the client faces dynamic internal and external challenges throughout the health-related event. During this time, both client and nurse undertake their own complex range of activities. These are listed in Table 30.

There is no one-to-one link between the various activities which comprise the work of nurse and client. The work of both is an integrated matrix in which each individual activity affects the whole. In each nursing encounter, the nurse selects from a full range of work strategies the most appropriate combination of actions to assist the client to progress through the passage.

The Work of the Client

The work the client seeks to accomplish during the passage arises from the total situation. It falls within the Nursing Partnership because nursing has strategies available to assist the client with this work.

Four major constructs were generated from the data to describe the major areas in the work of the client associated with negotiating the Nursing Partnership: Managing Self, Surviving the Ordeal, Affiliating with Experts, and Interpreting the Experience. Each one has a number of subconcepts.

TABLE 30: Negotiating the Nursing Partnership

The Work of the Client

Managing Self	Affiliating with Experts
Centring on Self	Acquiescing to Expertise
Harnessing Resources	Fitting In
Maintaining Equanimity	Retaining Autonomy
Surviving the Ordeal	Interpreting the Experience
Enduring Hardship	Monitoring Events
Tolerating Uncertainty	Developing Expertise
Possessing Hope	

The Work of the Nurse

Attending	Enabling
Being Present	Coaching
Ministering	Conserving
Listening	Extending
Comforting	Harmonising
	Encouraging

Interpreting
Responding
Anticipating

Managing Self

The client uses methods learned since childhood to prepare for and endure the experiences associated with a health-related event. This work has three identifiable subconcepts:

Centring on Self – the focus on self which permits the client make the most of the available energy to get through the present experience;

Harnessing Resources – the client's efforts to focus available resources as much as possible and to use learned self-management strategies to cope with each moment of the passage; and

Maintaining Equanimity – the client's work to attain a state of composure, serenity and quietude within, including a perceived need to present an acceptable face to others.

Affiliating with Experts

During a health-related event, a client may receive specialised assistance from a number of experts. In order to get the greatest benefit from this, the client has to learn strategies for interacting with these health personnel. Three subconcepts amplify the dimensions of this task:

Acquiescing to Expertise – the selective submission of the client to the experts on whose specialised skill and knowledge the person is now dependent;

Fitting In – the willingness, and ability, of the client to adapt to the routines and practices associated with receiving health care in any setting and to cooperate with nursing and other experts; and

Retaining Autonomy – the client's selective retention of independence in thought and action while receiving care from experts.

Surviving the Ordeal

The client works to endure the various experiences. There are three aspects to this work:

Enduring Hardship – the efforts made by the client to withstand experiences such as pain, discomfort and inconvenience;

Tolerating Uncertainty – the actions taken by the client to cope with the lack of certainty about such issues as the nature of the problem and the outcome of intervention, as well as the client's lack of specialised knowledge which limits the ability to make decisions concerning self and circumstances; and

Possessing Hope – the client's ability to anticipate a future in which there is an improvement in his or her condition and/or circumstances, which may be minutes, hours, days or even weeks away.

Interpreting the Experience

This construct continues the work of analysing events as they occur and synthesising them into a whole which has personal meaning. In addition to the constant processing of experiences and information, the client begins to use an increasing body of knowledge. This is reflected in two additional dimensions in the work:

Monitoring Events – the client uses an increasing knowledge base to form opinions on self-progress, the work of staff and occurrences in the environment; and

Developing Expertise – the client progressively processes information and becomes increasingly wise about the situation.

The Work of the Nurse

The negotiating work of the nurse is dynamic and sensitive as nursing strategies are selected and used to assist the client with his or her work at each stage. At any one time, a nursing action may encompass more than one type of nursing work in the way it is used to meet individual circumstances.

From the data, five theoretical constructs were developed to specify different aspects of nursing work: Attending, Enabling, Interpreting, Responding, and Anticipating.

Attending

Nursing work takes place during the moments of contact between nurse and client as the nurse accompanies the person through the experience of receiving health care. Thus, Attending denotes the first essential work of the nurse – being there for the person. It has four subconcepts:

Being Present – the spending of time with the client in order to nurse him or her in the immediacy of the ongoing passage;

Ministering – the selective application of nursing knowledge and skills to meet the identified needs of the client;

Listening – the concentration on what the client is saying and taking heed of this; and

Comforting – the effort made to soothe, ease any discomfort, and induce a state of well-being in a client.

Enabling

This is the empowering dimension of the nurse's work which assists the client to attain the means, opportunity and ability to act within the present circumstances. Five different subconcepts were identified within this construct:

Coaching – the guiding, motivating and teaching work of the nurse;

Conserving – the actions of the nurse which assist the client to protect, preserve and carefully manage available resources;

Extending – nursing's work to help the client to extend the scope of activities relevant to the current situation to enable the client to look after themselves as much as possible;

Harmonising – the help given to attain and/or maintain a beneficial state of harmony within the client or between the person and the environment; and

Encouraging – actions taken by the nurse to inspire a person with the confidence and the courage to hope, to grow, to take action, to make decisions, to accept help.

Interpreting

The nurse uses a number of methods to evaluate the status of the client and the situation. These include observing, monitoring, analysing, translating, contextualising, synthesising and decision-making. Interpreting – reasoning and judgement – exists as a separate planned activity during the appraising activities associated with entering and leaving the Nursing Partnership. It is also an integral part of every nursing action – a moment-by-moment activity as nursing continually adjusts to the client's evolving passage.

Responding

Throughout the partnership, the nurse is ready to take action in response to information received or to a perceived change in the client or his or her circumstances. This includes incidental responding at each nursing episode as well as planned, longer-term nursing responses.

Anticipating

The nurse is constantly challenged to use both knowledge and previous experience to visualise the client's immediate and/or longer-term future and to act to forestall a negative situation and/or help a beneficial outcome.

Leaving the Nursing Partnership

As the person's passage progresses, both client and nurse undertake new work to prepare the person for the transition from the Nursing Partnership. Time is a significant variable in this phase. There is an intrinsic sense of healing and progress which triggers the client to begin leaving preparations. In hospital the actual time for leaving hospital is usually decided by the medical staff, often in consultation with nurses. However, this may not be confirmed until the day of discharge. Thus, both client and nurse may have little time to complete their work if it is delayed until the actual time of discharge is confirmed.

In other nursing settings, and hopefully increasingly within the hospital, nursing criteria which relate to the client's readiness for leaving the Nursing Partnership will be valued, and the final decision will be a collaborative one between the client, the nursing and the medical staff.

The titles of the concepts within this phase remain unchanged and are listed on Table 31.

TABLE 31: Leaving the Nursing Partnership

The Work of the Client

Maximising Readiness
Making Arrangements
Discovering Requisites
Resuming Control

The Work of the Nurse

Appraising
Supplementing

The Work of the Client

The client engages in a number of tasks to prepare to leave the Nursing Partnership, and the care of a health agency. There are four separate but interrelated aspects to this work: Maximising Readiness, Making Arrangements, Discovering Requisites, and Resuming Control.

Making Arrangements

Prior to leaving the partnership, the client takes steps to prepare family and/or close friends for the upcoming departure and makes appropriate plans for actually going home if a change in setting is involved, as soon as the decision is made.

Discovering Requisites

The client needs to ascertain what measures are prescribed by members of the health-care team to continue progress after leaving the partnership.

Resuming Control

As the partnership draws to an end the client resumes self-care as much as possible, having shared this control with a number of experts during the passage.

The Work of the Nurse

During the Leaving phase, the nurse uses specific nursing strategies to ease the client's transition out of the Nursing Partnership as much as possible. Nursing is particularly concerned with ensuring that the person is as ready as possible to manage self-care, or receive appropriate assistance, on leaving the partnership. Two concepts were developed from the data to reflect the different aspects of the nurse's work at this time: Appraising and Supplementing.

Appraising

The nurse assesses the person's potential for self-care after leaving the partnership and identifies areas where immediate and longer-term support will be required. In this second formalised appraisal, the nursing staff use the Nursing Partnership model and a nursing appraisal of the client's status in concurrent passages, particularly medicine.

Supplementing

Following appraisal, the nurse arranges extra targeted assistance for the departing person. In negotiation with the client, arrangements are also made for future, specific assistance from nursing and other community services, if nursing judgement indicates this is a necessary adjunct to self and family care.

The Contextual Determinants

This aspect of the Nursing Partnership has undergone the greatest change. In the original model the contextual determinants were identified as those factors within the nursing context itself which exert a specific influence on the shape of the Nursing Partnership. However, it soon became clear that the model is incomplete without other contextual determinants which are equally significant in shaping each partnership. It is probable that others will be added as experience with the model in practice and education continues. Indeed, any group of nurses which plans to use the model is encouraged to reflect on the contextual determinants which are significant in their own particular area of nursing practice. Reflection on, and in-depth understanding of, these determinants is largely the professional responsibility of nurses before initiating a Nursing Partnership so that they are sensitive to their impact while working in partnership with each person.

At the present time the contextual determinants have been grouped into four categories consistent with the model: Within the Community, Within the Client, Within the Partnership, and Within the Nurse. They are summarised in Table 32.

TABLE 32: Contextual Determinants

Within the Community
Culture: Materials, Practices, Beliefs and Values
Health-Care System

Within the Client
Causal
Environmental

Within the Nursing Partnership
Episodic Continuity
Anonymous Intimacy
Mutual Benevolence

Within the Nurse
Nursing Knowledge
Nursing Wisdom
Regulation of Nursing
Conditions of Service

Within the Community
Culture: Materials, Practices, Beliefs and Values

Culture is used in its anthropological sense as the sum total of the material and intellectual equipment with which a people 'satisfy their biological and social needs and adapt themselves to their environment' (Piddington, 1963, p 4). It includes all the modifications human beings have made to the natural environment such as houses, clothing, food production and technological developments. These are integrally linked to the social aspects of the culture – the knowledge of natural phenomena and processes, systems of political and economic organisation, rules of morality, law and social behaviour, and spiritual beliefs and practices (ibid, p 4).

Within a modern community, there are likely to be many peoples, each with their own culture. Every culture is inevitably modified by the experience of living close to, and among, other peoples, and sharing the same environment. In addition, the way in which the community which contains the mix of cultural groups operates, becomes, in a sense, another culture. Often this community culture is largely determined by the practices, beliefs and values of the most powerful group. For example, within New Zealand there are a large number of cultures, but many of the integrating national materials, practices, beliefs and values have their roots in the white, British tradition. However, in their translation to a new setting, these aspects have been significantly modified by local factors, which includes the presence of the tangata whenua. The New Zealand national culture is continuing to change and develop in this way.

Each nurse has a responsibility to be culturally safe, that is, to know enough about the national and specific group cultures within the community to be able to nurse people, families and groups with sensitivity and without harm to their cultural identity.

Of particular importance are the beliefs and practices associated with health and well-being, with illness and disability, with the management of health-related experiences, and with life transitions such as birth and death which are held by the members of each group.

Both nurse and client are cultural beings. Nurses need to reflect on their own cultural selves and recognise that culture has a powerful impact on the behaviour of both participants working within a Nursing Partnership.

Health-Care System

The health-care system includes the range of services a community makes available to promote, maintain and protect the health of the people and to care for them when health-related problems occur. These services, which incorporate the community's beliefs about health and health care as well as the available financing, technology and trained health personnel, vary considerably from community to community. Nursing action is affected by the nature of the health-care system in several ways. Firstly, the nursing profession is usually the largest group within the system and its mode of operation is mainly prescribed by the resources, practices and beliefs influencing the provision of health care. Secondly, nursing staff are able to function more effectively within the Nursing Partnership if they are familiar with the services available to assist the people within the community.

Within the Client

Causal

This encompasses the range of human situations which may cause a person or group to require nursing. It is much more than the presence of a specifiable disease process with active medical intervention. Rather, it refers to the complex and unique human situations which result from the impact on the person and family of life experiences such as being born, dying, being ill, being disabled, suffering pain or despair, and seeking health. A person does not have to be sick in the medical sense to need nursing support. A Nursing Partnership focuses on the person and the nature of the work that person is being required to do to get through an event involving health. For example, a fragile elderly person may need intensive nursing and so might a mother with a new baby or a school-age child in need of health education.

Environmental

There is a complex matrix of physical, biological and sociocultural factors which influences each person and shapes behaviour during a health-related event. In addition to the person's cultural identity, these factors may range from living situation, climate, financial status, educational background, health history, physical state and many others.

Within the Nursing Partnership

Episodic Continuity

This is the paradox in which nursing is perceived as being continuous although, on examination, nursing is revealed as a series of episodes in which the nurse and client come into contact for only short periods of time for a specific purpose.

Anonymous Intimacy

In this second paradox, nursing is characterised by a degree of sanctioned closeness despite the fact that patient/clients are usually nursed by a constantly changing group of nurses, and nurses are faced with an ever-changing group of clients.

Mutual Benevolence

This construct refers to the reciprocal goodwill with which both client and nurse enter the Nursing Partnership, and which each seeks to maintain throughout the relationship.

Within the Nurse

Nursing Knowledge

The current body of nursing knowledge, skills and attitudes available to guide the nurse within the Nursing Partnership.

Nursing Wisdom

The sum total of the nursing education and practice experience of each nurse, and the accumulated nursing wisdom which guides the behaviour of the nurse.

Regulation of Nursing

The social requisites – sanctioned by local law and custom – which determine the scope of nursing practice and prescribe the behaviour required from individual nurses within a given community.

Conditions of Service

The employment conditions which determine the nature of the work environment for the nurse.

In this chapter the revised theoretical framework of the Nursing Partnership has been presented. As previously stated, it is a developing theory and further changes will take place. Nurses who are thinking of using the model are encouraged to experiment with the model and use their experience to modify it so that it works for them.

10   USING THE MODEL IN NURSING PRACTICE

As a field study which used qualitative methodology, the research which led to the Nursing Partnership produced data on both the problems and strengths of nursing practice in the surgical setting. Thus, the possibilities for nursing practice arise as much from an increased awareness and understanding of some of the problems as from the Nursing Partnership theory itself.

So often, while in the field and while analysing the data, the author was confronted with evidence that nursing could be piecemeal, disjointed, ritualised, lacking in both on-the-spot judgement and an integrating theoretical base. A significant number of nurses demonstrated either an inability or an unwillingness to complete a formalised nursing assessment on admission, few 'nursing problems' were identified, lists of disparate nursing directives were incomplete and inconsistently maintained. There was evidence that attention was given only to the task at hand. The recording of nursing care tended to be disjointed and often failed to reflect the process of nursing judgement. In fact, nursing records were consistently perceived as fulfilling an administrative requirement rather than actually helping the work of colleagues and easing the client's progress. Few oral or written comments linked nursing performance with a client response. Finally, there was an absence of formalised nursing-oriented discharge planning prior to the medical decision to send a person home.

Such comments may seem harsh but they reflect the field reality. However, as would be expected, there were also moments of excellence, some evidence of continuity, many episodes of nursing judgement and insight and safe nursing care. All these led to the creation of the grounded theory. The Nursing Partnership is not a panacea for the problems which currently exist in nursing practice. However, it does offer a fresh perspective on the processes involved in the giving and receiving of nursing.

Analysis of the field data revealed that nurses do possess or could attain the knowledge and skills that would permit the

Nursing Partnership as the theoretical basis for nursing practice. What nurses require is a guiding theoretical framework. Without this, nursing will remain undervalued, and consequently its perceived scope and function will be limited.

In this brief discussion on the possible implications of the Nursing Partnership perspective for nursing practice, several issues will be raised: conflict between ideal and reality, delivery of care, retention of qualified staff, nursing's focus on the person, nursing protocols and documentation, collegiality, quality assurance, and inservice education. Many of these issues have already been discussed in Chapter 2 and will not be repeated at this time.

Conflict Between Ideal and Real

The Nursing Partnership arises from nursing in practice. Thus, there should be an easier fit between the ideal and the real world of nursing. If the model is used in practice and in education, there would be a better opportunity to ally practice and education than presently is often the case.

However, nurses in practice often decry both the 'ideal' and those whom they perceive to be seeking to translate this into practice. The author can remember listening to a conversation among fellow students about a young capable nurse tutor where the greatest criticism was that she had performed nursing skills as a staff nurse in the way she had been taught – a major crime! Retention of an ideal/real dichotomy is not helpful. Rejection of the perceived ideal as unattainable tends to stultify nursing practice. If the ideal is not possible, then quality performance is not sought. Minimal performance persists. Poor performance may be repeated over and over again.

In the Nursing Partnership there is no ideal/real dichotomy. It is a theory that focuses on the possible. Optimal outcomes are negotiated in the context of complex realities. The nurse is constantly challenged to think, make choices, to negotiate, to challenge, to monitor self.

Delivery of Care

Over the years a number of strategies for the delivery of nursing care have been developed. Until recently these have tended to focus on the delivery of care over one eight-hour nursing shift. Task assignment was appropriate when nursing care was provided by a mixed team of student nurses and/or unqualified staff under the direct or indirect supervision of a registered nurse. Team nursing often meant task assignment but with a smaller number of nurses and clients. This could mean closer contact and more continuity of personnel. Cubicle nursing brought the possibility of even more contact as, theoretically, only one or two nurses might be involved in the care of the people within a room in a nursing unit.

Recently, the primary nursing model brought a dramatic change in the delivery of nursing care. In this model, the focus is on the client's total experience, not the eight-hour shift. A designated primary nurse, acceptable to the client, has 24-hour responsibility for the care of a person for the duration of that person's need for nursing. Thus, the primary nurse combines decision-making with bedside care. In practice, many have interpreted this model as giving all the responsibility to the primary nurse and none to the registered nurses who care for the person when the primary nurse is not on duty – 'He's not my patient. I just do what I'm told.' This interpretation is possible if accountability for decision-making is only visible at the level of the primary nurse. However, such a view is not consistent with the use of the Nursing Partnership.

The Nursing Partnership theory requires accountability at the individual level. In a team of registered nurses, the primary nursing model has value but requires modification. Instead of requiring primary nurses to leave behind a set of 'instructions' to which others must adhere in their absence, an amended model would see the primary nurse as the coordinator of a nursing partnership with a responsibility to guide and monitor the evolving passage (Manthey, 1980, p 33). Each nurse giving care to a particular client is accountable for on-the-spot nursing judgements and action, in a professional sense, to the primary nurse who is responsible for overall outcome and nursing action. This would decentralise quality assurance from a specialist department to the team of practising nurses within a nursing unit. Thus the mode of nursing-care delivery, the theoretical framework for practice and quality control would be in synchrony.

Retention of Qualified Staff

In the light of the prevailing concern for the loss of experienced nursing staff from practice through attrition, or their replacement with unqualified staff, there is a need for nurses to have the confidence that comes from a framework for nursing practice that clearly asserts nursing's contribution to health care. This assertion must be in word and in deed. Quality nursing practice and increased job satisfaction are urgently needed.

This challenge is given some urgency by the findings of a recent case study of seven local nurses who have left nursing. The researcher, herself a nurse, reached a sobering conclusion.

> The women in this study had, for the sake of a better word, simply 'outgrown' the system. They had outgrown it in terms of their clinical work. Nursing was unable to provide for them sufficient advancement opportunities, sufficient intellectual stimulation or sufficient responsibility to warrant staying in their hospital jobs. In their development as women they also had outgrown the system. They had developed a sense of their own value which made working in a system that demanded more than it gave, unrealistic for today's society. The demand is for a dedication and commitment, and the rewards are inequality in the workplace, undervalued work, and long, difficult and inconvenient working hours. There are no easy solutions to these complex problems but perhaps it is time for another reassessment of nursing . . . . It is also time to address the nineteenth century problem of the 'subservience of nurses' that has relentlessly plagued nursing through this century and from which stem many of today's problems. (Paterson, 1989, p 37)

Excellence, borne of the wisdom of education and experience, needs to be recognised and rewarded. Nurses, colleagues and employers should be encouraged to support those who demonstrate expertise in their practice. It is easy to agree with Benner, who writes that the encouragement of excellence in nursing practice is significant for the future of nursing.

> Expertise in complex decision-making, such as nursing requires, makes the interpretation of clinical situations possible, and the knowledge embedded in this clinical expertise is central to the advancement of nursing practice and the development of nursing science. (Benner, 1984, p 3)

The Nursing Partnership perspective supports this goal by encouraging this kind of performance by the registered nurse. When using the theoretical approach in practice, each nurse making a contribution to a client's passage would be required to be open to the client's ongoing experience. The nurse would enter each Nursing Partnership, and each nursing encounter within an ongoing partnership, aware that the model offers a constant opportunity to use the full range of available nursing resources to progress the client through a passage. Individual nursing episodes are essentially private transactions, and so supporting the commitment of all nurses to seek excellence in their own practice – and consequently supporting quality collaborative work by the nursing team – becomes a prerequisite for an effective qualified work-force.

Focus on the Person

The Nursing Partnership focuses on the total experience of a person involved in a health-related event. It is a model which allows the nurse to care for a person and to practise primary health care at all times. A medical problem and its intervention, if present, are significant but not the sole determinants of nursing care. This perspective releases the nurse from any suggested subservience to medicine and gives her a means by which to clearly articulate nursing's specific contribution to care in any situation.

Nursing Protocols and Documentation

At this point, it is important to state that the Nursing Partnership is proposed as a theoretical framework for use by registered nurses. As such, it is not proposed to offer specific practice protocols and associated forms of documentation – nursing history, nursing care plan, etc. Rather, it would be expected that any nurses considering using the approach in practice would, first of all, familiarise themselves with the model. Then, as a groups of experts in their own nursing practice setting, they would make any required adjustments and use their collective nursing wisdom to develop the appropriate practice protocols and documentation to guide its use. There needs to be an ongoing process of collaboration and review to ensure that developed practice protocols remain relevant.

In practice, if nursing histories are used to guide information gathering, they often take the form of checklists of incidental information which lack an integrating framework to give them purpose. In this way they fail to get the kind of information that is needed to found subsequent nursing practice. Within the Nursing Partnership framework, particular attention is given to the client's prelude experience. A specific theoretical shape has been assigned to it. Nursing significance is attached to the person's experience of living with a health-related problem and its consequences over a period of time. This total experience has a complex and significant impact on the person, on their work and thus on the Nursing Partnership. The patterned Beginning provides a framework which helps the nurse to gather knowledge about the critical areas of the client's prelude which will be relevant to the client's nursing.

During the transition phase into the Nursing Partnership, nurses are able to use the model to orient their nursing work. The conceptualisation of the person's passage, the participants' mutual work, and the contextual determinants which influence the people and the partnership, guide the nurse through the open-ended discovery-oriented discussion which is a part of the initial formal nursing appraisal. By this means, a rich base of information which is relevant to nursing is available to nurses at the outset of a working partnership. As a consequence, nurses are able to use, and reuse, this information as they initiate appropriate nursing strategies to ease the client's way through the passage.

A nursing care plan should be practical and useable. It must reflect the setting in which nursing is being practised. For example, the plan for a nursing team of qualified nurses will be different from that developed for a team which includes nursing assistants. The latter will contain more specific and detailed guidelines for care which permit untrained staff to implement care prescribed by the supervising registered nurse. By contrast, the former will focus on broad concepts which guide and coordinate nursing behaviour within each partnership, and recognise the need for the autonomous, mutually accountable performance of each member of the nursing team. Benner found that 'the expert nurse can interpret particular situations and make the necessary exceptions and alterations in the rules in order to individualise patient care' (ibid, p 176). Thus, a nursing approach which has an associated documentation format that both requires and enables the registered nurse to practise on-the-spot decision-making, supported by cues recorded from previous nursing episodes, will encourage professional accountability and responsibility. This behaviour is self-evident within the Nursing Partnership.

As the passage progresses, the changing pattern of the client's work, together with any available medical and related information, would prompt the nurse to recognise that the client is entering into the Leaving phase. At this time a protocol is required to guide the registered nurse to begin to assist the person to prepare for this transition experience.

The Nursing Partnership may be a helpful conceptual framework for professional practice because it permits, indeed encourages, the continuous inclusion of new knowledge and technology without threatening the overall approach to nursing practice.

Collegiality

This theoretical approach requires nurses to adopt a collegial partnership in which autonomous nurses work together, each making a valuable contribution to the progress of a single Nursing Partnership – building on what has gone before, contributing to what is to come. Through such partnerships, nursing is translated into action 24 hours a day as many parallel passages take their course. This approach would preclude the perception of nursing as a continuing private transaction between one nurse and one client, even during the one nursing shift. As this study has shown, it is the norm that nursing is one nurse with many clients; many clients with one nurse.

While addressing a nursing symposium, a doctor made a comment which demonstrates that even the people who supposedly work alongside nurses may not recognise the significance of nursing's contribution to patient care.

> My personal journey as a partner of nurses really began when I was confronted by the realisation of a missing component in effective care. Competent assessment of problems and accurate prescription of appropriate therapy was not enough to make many of the persons I was caring for well. In the intervals between the medical decisions I made there was a whole world I knew little of – a gap in the care of and caring for patients and their families. The clinical work of my nursing colleagues filled that gap. (Hansen, 1979)

The Nursing Partnership, an integrated vision of nursing practice, can help nurses to articulate this 'missing component in effective care' for themselves, their clients and their colleagues. By linking each nursing action within a patterned and purposeful process, it may give nurses increased confidence to assert their role in the nursing-medical partnership.

Quality Assurance

It is possible that the Nursing Partnership could be used to generate criteria by which the effectiveness of nursing care could be judged.

The various dimensions of client and nurse behaviour and their place in the partnership could be used to develop nursing standards at the unit and professional level. In its modified form, the model could serve as a basis for the mutual sharing of nursing knowledge and experience between nurses working in a variety of practice settings. As such, it may provide a common language that could vitalise nursing within an organisation by stimulating the performance of individual nurses and increasing their commitment to their clients, to their colleagues, and to nursing. Also, such a concerted approach would encourage ongoing self and peer review associated with an articulated set of standards for nursing performance.

Inservice Education

Within the practice setting, staff education programmes seek to maintain a consistent quality of work performance from the nursing staff. This work is made more difficult by the mobile nature of the nursing work-force and the difficulty demonstrated in retaining expert nurses in hands-on nursing roles. One consequence is that priority is given to the continuous initiation of newly registered nurses into work settings where, by default, they may become the 'experts' in a matter of months as more experienced nurses leave. In this environment, there is a need for a career structure which encourages, identifies and rewards excellence in nursing practice using specific nursing criteria. This lack of a path for progression in nursing practice means there is an associated lack of developmental programmes which focus on the continuing development of registered nurses.

Even in its present stage of development, the Nursing Partnership has possibilities in the practice setting. It is a tool that nurses can use creatively in the mutual interests of nurse and client. The partnership model is also consistent with the expressed aspirations of the community.

11 USING THE MODEL IN NURSING EDUCATION

As they undertake the challenging work of developing curricula for courses leading to registration, nurses working in the field of education seek answers to a number of key questions.

- What should a nurse be able to do at the time of registration?
- How do people become nurses?
- What is the best way to assist the student who is making the transition from lay person to registered nurse?

These have never been easy questions to answer. They are even harder to answer today as dramatic political and social changes are occurring in most societies throughout the world. Naturally, events of this kind have a profound effect on nurses and the service they provide within their community. Courses of study which prepare registered nurses are affected by the state of the economy as well as changing philosophies and policies in education and health care. Other influences on nursing education come from the often conflicting expectations of the nursing profession, students, consumers of nursing care, potential employers and the community as a whole.

A consensual model for human relationships is gaining popularity in the wider community as well as in both education and health care. This is associated with the increased interest in issues such as equity, consumer and women's rights, individual responsibility and accountability. The concept of partnership fits in with this development.

This chapter introduces the concept of a Learning Partnership model which can be derived from the Nursing Partnership. Following this, the discussion focuses on a number of related issues: teacher-centred content or learner-centred process; developing independence; developing creativity; learning to contextualise nursing; nursing partnership as content; and teaching as exemplar of creativity with responsibility, independence and partnership.

The Learning Partnership

It is possible to translate the dimensions of the Nursing Partnership directly into a Learning Partnership. Learning can be perceived as an adventure in which the student becomes a nurse by exploring the complex terrain of nursing knowledge and practice, under the guidance of a nurse-teacher. The dimensions of experience, mutual work and context are present in both learning and nursing.

A curriculum based on the partnership model would describe the overall pattern for the learning experience associated with becoming a nurse. However, the teaching/learning philosophy supporting the Learning Partnership model would also articulate the school's commitment to supporting and encouraging individuality in each student's path to registration. At the outset, the teacher guides a process of negotiation in which both learner and teacher develop a common vision of the process and outcome of the partnership. This consensus is essential if both participants are to work harmoniously together to develop the student's potential to practise nursing in a way which combines skill and artistry.

Within the Learning Partnership model the nurse-teacher partner acts as a representative of nursing and teaching. Expertise in both areas is required to plan and participate in the integrated programme of incremental learning experiences which comprise the curriculum. These encourage and support every student's development of the abilities described in the graduate profile, namely, those of the beginning registered nurse.

During the pre-partnership phase the teacher works to maintain a readiness for teaching which includes preparation for the teaching role, knowledge of teaching and organisational protocols, and current subject knowledge. The transition experiences of entering and leaving are important stages in the partnership. Both participants work to ease the path for the learner. In the entry phase the teacher seeks to gain an understanding of the characteristics every student brings with them into the partnership, including cultural background, learning style, qualifications, experience and expectations. This insight into the learner is actively sought and valued by the teacher.

As proposed, the major areas of ongoing work of the student can also be classified into the four dimensions of managing self, affiliating with experts, surviving and interpreting the experience. Students work in these four areas as they use the time and resources available to engage in activities associated with the process of becoming a nurse. Thus, they explore the knowledge base of nursing practice; practise the wide range of skills required of the registered nurse; learn to value the individuality, complexity and integrity of each person; learn to combine reflection with practice; and develop the courage to challenge the continuing relevance of the status quo. A strong and independent nursing identity is emergent throughout the partnership.

As with nursing within the Nursing Partnership teaching is a dynamic, skilful activity. The teacher selectively uses strategies associated with attending, enabling, anticipating, responding and interpreting to guide and support the work of the student. Accumulated knowledge and skills are used creatively in a dynamic moment-by-moment decision-making process to facilitate student learning.

Every Learning Partnership is influenced by a range of contextual determinants which can be classified into four broad categories, namely, within the community, within the learner, within the teacher, and within the partnership. Any curriculum using a partnership model would seek to identify the characteristics of the environment. Both teacher and learner are sensitive to the way in which their relationship and their work is embedded in, and shaped by the context.

Teacher-Centred Content or Learner-Centred Process

Nursing curricula, like many in tertiary education, are often teacher-centred. Institution and teacher are clearly in control of the teaching process. Often, curricula literally bulge with content deemed to be essential by the teaching staff. More and more information may be added as nurse educators strive to meet the need to prepare large numbers of graduates who are capable of functioning at a beginning registered nurse level in every nursing setting – medical, surgical, psychiatric, psychopaedic, paediatric, obstetric, and geriatric as well as in the community.

Additional pressure can be placed on teachers to broaden curricula to include increasing amounts of knowledge drawn from the arts, humanities, social sciences, and physical and biological sciences. More recently, increasing sensitivity to the social and cultural differences which separate people and threaten the ability of nurses and clients to work together has led to calls for nursing students to be able to safely nurse a person from another culture. A common response is yet more courses such as social anthropology or transcultural nursing. Thus, more and more content is added.

It is common for a content-driven curriculum to be associated with an assembly-line model of teaching, with all students having a standardised set of learning experiences. The student's role is to be a sponge, absorbing the prescribed schedule of knowledge, skills and attitudes. Most teaching takes place in the anonymity of large groups. Evaluation frequently takes the form of mass, content-focused methods such as multichoice questions and essays. Usually, this approach is associated with an extremely tight time-frame for completion of the dual requirements for registration and a tertiary diploma or degree. Teachers face real conflict as they seek to balance the competing and often irreconcilable demands for mastery of theoretical content and the achievement of competence.

An alternative approach is a learner-centred curriculum based on a guiding philosophy which encourages the mutuality associated with a partnership approach. Learning to nurse can be viewed as a transition passage, a journey which takes students from the status of lay person at the point of entry into a programme to the exit stage when they are ready to assume the role of registered nurse. Abilities associated with the profile of the graduate are clearly identified. Learners accept the challenge of working their way towards achievement of a series of required learning outcomes, all of which contribute to the achievement of the graduate profile.

In such a curriculum learning is an asymmetrical partnership in which both learner and teacher focus on the student's ongoing experience. Both acknowledge that the experience of becoming a nurse is 'owned' by the student. Students take full responsibility for their own learning, while teachers use their specialised wisdom, borne of experience and education, to support them in that transforming process.

Developing Independence

In many countries health care delivery is being profoundly influenced by a management philosophy which includes a flattening of organisational structures and a commitment to the belief that every person must accept full accountability and responsibility for their own work. By philosophy, supervision is largely redundant and quality assurance is considered to be best maintained through self and peer review.

In this environment a separate nursing organisation with multi-level supervision of staff and practice is no longer sustainable. Indeed, the new management philosophy challenges nursing's traditional view of itself, its governance of nursing care and its place in the health care team. Now, management of nursing personnel is being separated from the management of nursing practice. In many areas there is a marked reduction in senior nursing management. Roles such as Director of Nursing, Nursing Supervisor and Charge Nurse are being reviewed and often abandoned. Each nurse is required to be responsible for self.

At the same time, new practice opportunities are becoming available. Independent practice is now much more common. More than ever before the profession requires nursing education programmes to produce skilful, resourceful, independent practitioners with a strong nursing identity who are well-grounded in their knowledge of self and others. They need a sense of confidence in their ability to nurse people in the complex reality of their life experiences, regardless of the setting. Situation-specific nursing judgement requires the creative and selective application of every nurse's accumulated body of nursing knowledge and skills. A spirit of inquiry characterises this new nursing practice.

Nursing education has been influenced by the public investigation of events involving the practice of health professionals. In New Zealand, for example, nurses in both practice and education have been challenged to rethink how students are socialised into nursing by the comments of Judge Sylvia Cartwright. Following an extended period of investigation into a research programme involving women with cervical carcinoma in situ at National Women's Hospital in the 1960s she found it necessary to comment on her perception of the behaviour of nurses – past and present.

> Nurses have been conditioned to protect patients by stealth. They cannot therefore be effective advocates who will act bravely and independently. (Cartwright, 1988, p 173)

How can nurses in education respond to this comment made by a respected lawyer? 'Brave and independent' nurses require a strong sense of self-identity, an ability to articulate a nursing viewpoint appropriately and convincingly, and an ability to fulfil the requirements of being a full member of a collegial health care team. Each member of this team has a socially sanctioned responsibility to protect the community from harm.

Buckenham and McGrath also challenge nurses in practice and education when, at the conclusion of a study involving in-depth interviews with students and nurses in Australia, they state that

> . . . if nurses, as students, are subjected to a system which demands deferential and subordinate behaviour, which teaches them to consider themselves subservient, and which insists that they view the patient as external, if not inferior, to the health team, is it any wonder that, after registration, that nurses display those same characteristics? After three years of practising those behaviours and internalising those attitudes, surely it is unreasonable to expect them to perform in any other way. (Buckenham and McGrath, 1983, p 105)

While the curriculum alone cannot encourage the student to attain and maintain a strong independent nursing identity, this should now be a major focus of any nursing education programme.

Students enter a programme with varying levels of self-knowledge, independent learning, and strategies for supplementing personal resources in times of need. Some may not possess these abilities to the level required to participate in the Learning Partnership as described. These students require considerable specialised teaching support to attain them. Independence and self-knowledge are both required and constantly encouraged throughout the student's personal experience of becoming a nurse.

Developing Creativity through Partnership

A learner-centred curriculum emphasises discovery and critical thinking, and rejects the suggestion that nursing can be routinised into a set of known rules and procedures to be learned by rote. There is a need for teaching staff to create learning opportunities which closely link discovery and critical thinking with the development of accountability in the learner for both autonomous and collaborative action. Throughout each learning experience students need to have opportunities to challenge, to seek clarification when uncertain, to make choices, to learn to negotiate with teachers, nurses in practice and clients, to give reasons for decisions, to evaluate self, to value critical review, to give thoughtful feedback and to review negotiated goals.

In the laboratory and practice settings students also need to be able to practise making decisions, and to justify them when challenged by teachers and peers. Self and peer review are critical behaviours which the student is assisted to master during the learning process. This requirement arises from the belief that the ability to be accountable and to accept personal responsibility for one's own behaviour are valued characteristics of a graduating nurse.

Students learn to balance creative decision-making with risk in situations where peoples' lives are involved. Mistakes will occur, and must be permitted, as the student learns. Nurse educators are required to exercise considerable wisdom in their responses to important questions. How much simulated learning will take place before the student is exposed to the 'real-life' situation? How closely will the student be supervised? How will the teacher encourage the learner to make choices? How will mistakes be managed? How will the partnership between teacher and an independent learner develop? The way teachers manage these issues will provide exemplars to the students of behaviour that demonstrates both creativity and responsibility.

As the Learning Partnership progresses, students also benefit from an association with expert nurses who demonstrate excellence in the creative application of nursing knowledge and skill as they work in partnership with clients in 'the real world' of nursing practice. Role-modelling in the context of the everyday world of nursing practice is invaluable. Exemplar nurses in practice have a profound effect on the student's experience of becoming a nurse. A series of planned encounters with experienced practitioners and/or lecturer/practitioners presents the student with a reality-based understanding of the boundaries and possibilities of nursing action.

Learning to Contextualise Nursing

Any curriculum using a partnership model for both learning and nursing cannot simultaneously adopt a positivist model for the presentation of content. This approach requires the learner to systematically study a range of phenomena, which are assumed to behave according to universal laws. From this perspective there is a decontextualised, linear relationship between cause and effect. Indeed, everything can be explained and prediction is reliable. If this were the case, nursing could be organised into a set of prescribed responses to common situations, with predictable outcomes.

By contrast, the partnership model represents both nursing and learning as highly contextualised activities. Each nursing and learning encounter involves a complex and unique blending of multidimensional factors arising within the partners, the relationship and the context. There is no simple linear path between cause, effect, response and outcome. Instead, complexity and uncertainty prevail. Each situation shares its building blocks with others, but the way the blocks are put together reflects the particular blend of circumstances which have come together.

Every day nurses in practice face new human situations they have not encountered before. To prepare for this, students need to develop the ability to identify individual patterns and to select between multiple probabilities in a creative way. By requiring students to pose questions, search for evidence, identify options, exercise judgement, take action, and assess outcomes, teachers guide the establishment of a personal database which will prepare the graduate for the reality of nursing practice.

Contextualisation is further enhanced by an openness between student and teacher which encourages exploration of the multiple dimensions which are influencing the Learning Partnership itself. Students become aware of the many determinants which are shaping their own journey. Through this process students are sensitised to the embedding of partnerships in context, and will be able to transfer this awareness to their nursing practice.

Nursing Partnership as Content

Nurse educators face the challenge of developing curricula with a nursing framework which has a comfortable fit for the selection and organisation of selected knowledge from medical science as well as the biological, physical and social sciences, and the humanities. Students need to understand the reason for learning this related knowledge. Protests by some students that they do not want to become 'mini' doctors or scientists, or by other students that they do not have enough of this related content, both need to be addressed when they occur. It is important for the curriculum to require students to use knowledge drawn from other disciplines in combination with nursing knowledge.

The way in which curriculum content is organised can serve to reinforce nursing as either an assistive, dependent job or an autonomous profession with a distinctive body of knowledge. At the present time there are few effective theoretical frameworks which give a strong nursing focus. Consequently, many nurses feel that increasing their 'medical' knowledge is the only way to make them 'better' nurses. It is possible that the Nursing Partnership could minimise the prevalence of this belief by replacing it with a perspective which values related knowledge as complementary and supportive to a strongly independent form of nursing practice. Emphasis would then be placed on the reality that nursing's mission is to work with people to enhance their well-being during a health-related event.

Each teaching team has to reach a consensus decision on the way nursing knowledge will be presented in a curriculum. Students need to have an opportunity to critically examine nursing's body of knowledge. The use of the Nursing Partnership as the theoretical framework for nursing encourages a research-derived division into parts, namely the multiple dimensions of people who become patient/clients, a nursing perspective on health-related human experiences, the work of the nurse, relationships and the context of nursing practice. This model also provides an integrative framework for drawing these parts into a whole. Choices on the way the partnership model could be used in a nursing curriculum are limited only by the imagination and wisdom of the collegial team of teachers within a nursing department, and by the collective strength of their own nursing identity.

Teaching as Exemplar of Creativity with Responsibility, Independence and Partnership

Within any nursing curriculum a group of nurse teachers work with colleagues from a variety of disciplines to offer a nursing programme. They are required to demonstrate many of the same qualities as they require in the students. The curriculum philosophy, framework, principles and goals are established within a collegial team.

The curriculum is not developed to a stage where each teacher is given a detailed teaching programme which must be taught exactly as prescribed. This would be the antithesis of the kind of autonomous professional practice – incorporating collegiality, independent judgement, responsibility and the creative application of knowledge to individual situations – which is required from both teacher and nurse today.

Instead, the curriculum includes a clearly articulated profile of the graduate supported by a teaching/learning climate which is in tune with the outcome. Each member of the teaching team is required to be in agreement, and completely familiar, with the curriculum framework and the teacher/learning philosophy. They use their own expertise to develop teaching programmes which actualise the curriculum.

Professional behaviour is demonstrated in each teacher's role as partner within the learning partnership. There is continuing accountability for personal and group decisions and actions to colleagues, to students, to nurse colleagues in practice, and to the community through the processes of accreditation and moderation. Thus, each teacher becomes a highly visible model as personal teaching and nursing wisdom are creatively harnessed to support student learning throughout the partnership.

Summary

There is no doubt that a state of turbulence exists in the delivery of health care and in the role of the nurse throughout the world. It is essential for nurses in education, in collaboration with colleagues from service, to develop programmes which will prepare beginning registered nurses for the reality of nursing practice today, and with the potential to respond to the challenges they will meet in the health care system of tomorrow.

The partnership model could be of assistance in nursing education in two ways. Firstly, it could provide the shape for the learning/ teaching process through which the transformation into registered nurse takes place. Secondly, it could be used as the professional nursing framework for the organisation of content within the curriculum. Thus, complementary partnership models for teaching and nursing would work together to guide the complex process of learning to nurse.

[1] This quote has been amended to remove the authors' use of female pronouns.

12   THE FUTURE

The Nursing Partnership, in its original form, has been systematically described. All constituent elements within the grounded theory have been introduced and discussed with the field data from which they emerged. The concept results from the creative induction processes associated with the grounded theory method. Using the terminology of this method, it is a grounded theory in discussional form which awaits further development to the propositional form. At present, it is a theoretical framework and, as such, a theory in the process of development.

The setting, five surgical wards in a large general hospital, was a complex and challenging field for research. For the nursing staff, it is the workplace where they nurse within a team of qualified nurses. For the patients, it is the place where problems are made better by surgical means, and this brings them into contact with nursing. This research was initiated to formulate an interpretation of the transaction between nurse and client while the latter is in hospital. The question was posed: What is happening here? The response was a conceptualisation of the giving and receiving of nursing as a partnership – the Nursing Partnership.

After the research was completed, the theory continued its development. Comments from colleagues and the experience of working with the model in a new curriculum led to reflection and change. A revised version of the Nursing Partnership has been presented and its constituent elements defined. This revision tended to generalise the model's applicability so that nurses in other settings can use it. The contentious issue of which term to use – 'patient' or 'client' – was resolved by using the term 'client', while recommending that those using the model feel free to use the term most appropriate for their use. A nursing prelude was also added and recognition was given to the broad range of contextual determinants which have an impact on the Nursing Partnership.

Possible use of the theoretical framework in nursing practice and education has been discussed briefly.

There is a need to continue to develop the theory from its present stage to a set of propositions which deal with relationships on a variety of levels. Explanatory and predictive statements are required. These could arise as hypotheses based on the many relationships implied in the findings of this study.

One research of major significance would be a study of the theory's use in practice and in education. In practice, this would require a nursing unit to decide to use it and set up a study to evaluate its impact on clients, nurses and the unit. Individual passages and partnerships could be examined and analysed in detail. Such a study would clarify the relationship between nursing action and client behaviour. Facilitating and non-facilitating nurse actions associated with each area of client work could be identified in the context of the partnership. Indicators of nursing effectiveness in progressing a client through a passage are required as well as a set of diagnostic criteria to assist the nurse to judge the immediate and continuing effectiveness of the work of the clients within the circumstances of their situation.

In education, any school that develops a curriculum based on the model has an obligation to monitor the outcome from an educational and practice perspective. The refinements to the model to date have come from the reflective suggestions of nurse educators.

In essence, further research on the grounded theory of the Nursing Partnership is dependent on the imagination of those who wish to investigate it. There are many possibilities.

After a study of this kind, in which a large topic has been examined using a creative methodology, much remains unsaid. The work remains incomplete. During the course of the analysis, many worthwhile avenues of inquiry opened and were then discarded as the decision was made to concentrate on developing the Nursing Partnership. Alternative perspectives on the data remain unexplored. However, the study has generated a perspective on nursing which challenges nurses to reflect on their practice.

This journey of discovery has been interrupted to write this book, to share the emerging grounded theory in its present form. The effort has been and continues to be worthwhile because nursing really can make a difference. The journey will continue.

Hopefully others in nursing, having read this, will feel it belongs to them and will share in its further development.

He waka eke noa.
A canoe on which everyone may embark.

APPENDIX 1
The Research Method

Over recent years there has been increasing interest in the use of qualitative research methods to study nursing. Justification for this approach can take the form of criticism of quantitative methods and/or espousal of the cause of qualitative methodology. Elements of both approaches will be apparent in the discussion that follows. However, advocacy for qualitative field research, and the grounded theory method in particular, is limited to its appropriateness for this study and the resolution of the questions with which the researcher was concerned. Thus the value of the approach is emphasised, and care has been taken to avoid involvement in the general area of criticism of methodologies which has become a 'well-established form of professional recreation' (Hill, 1970, p 16).

This study was planned to be an exploration of nursing in the hospital setting. There would be no manipulation of events, no experimentation, and no predetermined hypotheses. Rather, the researcher set out to enter the natural setting ready to observe and to attach meaning to what happens when a patient is being nursed through the experience of planned surgery.

> . . . to discover the elusive, vague, and still largely unexplored nature of human care necessitates exquisite participant observations, interviews, documentations, and other research skills and techniques mainly associated with qualitative types of research. (Leininger, 1985, p xi)

All of these strategies were used to gather data from the experiences of patients and nurses as they interact in 'the private, intimate world of human care' (Watson, 1985b, p 345). The question to be posed in this field was: What is happening here? Such a question involves the researcher fully in the process of data gathering and analysis and the consequent induction of a meaningful interpretation of what is happening. The grounded theory approach to the discovery of theory was chosen as the most suitable method for this field research.

The following discussion on the research method has been organised under three headings: Qualitative Research in Nursing, The Nurse as Researcher, and The Grounded Theory Method.

Qualitative Research in Nursing

Qualitative research permits the researcher to explore a problem area in its natural setting. Support for the use of a qualitative method suggests it allows the researcher to 'move close to a social setting and bring back an accurate picture of patterns and phenomenological reality as they are experienced by human beings in social capacities' (Lofland, 1971, p 59).

Nursing is concerned with 'the dynamic whole that is a human being with whom the nurse interacts in practice' (Omery, 1983, p 49). There is a recognition that multiple and complex phenomena are operating in the transaction between nurse and patient. Identification and description of each is possible, but their interrelatedness is an essential component of a theoretical representation of the reality of nursing.

Further support for the consistency between a qualitative approach and the focus of concern of nursing comes from Tinkle and Beaton.

> At its most basic level, nursing is a relational profession. It exists by virtue of its commitment to provide care to others. If the concerns and perceptions of the recipients of nursing services are considered unimportant factors in nursing research, then nurses may indeed be providing nursing care that is more meaningful to themselves than to patients. (Tinkle and Beaton, 1983, p 31)

This view is shared by Munhall when she proposes that:

> . . . qualitative research methods, particularly in theory development, may be more consistent with nursing's stated philosophical beliefs in which subjectivity, shared experience, shared language, interrelatedness, human interpretation, and reality as experienced rather than contrived are considered. (Munhall, 1982, p 178)

The final example of support for a qualitative approach to be introduced comes from Swanson and Chenitz who, after defining qualitative research as 'a systematic study of the world of everyday experience', go on to state:

> Qualitative research provides a way to construct meaning that is more reflective of the world of practice because its methodology, like its subject, is more organic than mechanistic and, therefore, more suitable to the domain of professional nursing. Scientific discovery in nursing will come with the generation of theory that explains client situations from a perspective that is uniquely our own. Qualitative research provides avenues for these discoveries. (Swanson and Chenitz, 1982, p 245)

With the goal of the research being the discovery of new insights, the outcome is uncertain during much of the process. The reseacher must remain open to the significance of the data despite the possibility of moments of panic when facing masses of data with no outcome in sight. The presence and validity of such a feeling is confirmed by Deutscher.

> It is scary because the research outcomes are unpredictable. The nightmare of every qualitative researcher, novice or experienced, is 'What if I don't

find anything?' The fact that one is always able to find something because there is always something there is not reassuring. (Deutscher, 1975, p vi)

However, two previous experiences of fieldwork using qualitative methodologies had prepared the researcher for the challenges inherent in the use of such a research approach (Christensen 1971; 1972). In-depth analysis of the nursing literature reaffirmed the value of using a discovery method to answer the broad research question: What is happening here?

The Nurse as Researcher

The use of a qualitative method involves entry into the field to gather data on the experiences of people as they occur. Therefore, the researcher becomes a participant and does have an impact on people and events. The degree of influence depends on the extent and type of participation by the researcher in the field. Four distinct roles, each of which is characterised by a different mix of observation and participation, have been suggested by Junker and these can be summarised as follows:

1 *Complete Participant* – here the researcher becomes a complete member of the group under study and observational activities are completely concealed from the members of the group.

2 *Participant as Observer* – the researcher does not totally conceal observation activities, but such activities are subordinated to participation activities which give the researcher entry to the field.

3 *Observer as Participant* – the observation activities are publicly known from the beginning and sanctioned by those in the field, giving the researcher access to the field but perhaps influencing the 'openness' of members in giving information to the researcher.

4 *Complete Observer* – an almost imaginary role in which the researcher has complete freedom to observe without any influence on the activities or group under study. (Junker, 1960, pp 35–38)

In this study, the role adopted by the researcher was primarily that of 'observer as participant'. There was full disclosure to all concerned that a research project was underway and that the researcher was a nurse herself. As a nurse, the researcher was familiar with the setting. In this respect, the nature of the research is different from that in which a social scientist enters a field with which that person has had no previous experience.

Nursing needs nurses as researchers in order to ask and investigate the questions of significance to the profession (Schlotfeldt, 1972, p 484). However, the role of nurse researcher in a field study is not an easy one.

. . . being a nurse and a researcher can present difficulties, especially when the researcher explores nursing problems by participant-observation. How does the nurse researcher live with both halves of her hyphenated self as she studies practice in the only place it can be studied, the field of practice? (McBride, Diers and Schmidt, 1970, p 1256)

On the one hand, the nurse researcher may avoid the '"culture shock" experienced by a non-nurse on entry to the field' and may be 'sensitive to certain aspects of nursing behaviour which a non-nurse may not notice' (Byerly, 1976, p 148). Conversely, the nurses' professional orientation may confine their 'openness' to what is happening as they interpret events and the data within an a priori framework. In addition, nursing experience may lead to the researcher being used by subjects as a 'source of advice on how to solve problems', 'a sounding board, and sometimes as an object of catharsis' (ibid, p 149). Despite potential difficulties, advocates for increasing the use of qualitative research in nursing suggest that the nurse researcher should acknowledge the value of the joint role and, indeed, use it to enhance the quality of the research (Quint, 1969; Fagerhaugh and Strauss, 1977).

Entry into the field to collect data does mean that the researcher becomes involved in the everyday life of the people involved. Relationships develop between the researcher and the people in the setting which will influence the study. According to Zigarmi and Zigarmi, both subject and researcher can feel the unidirectionality of the relationship if the researcher is 'always taking' and the subject 'always giving' (Zigarmi and Zigarmi, 1979, p 26). The subject will be interested in the research activities and, therefore, it is important for the researcher to accept the responsibility of reciprocating on a person-to-person basis (Wax, 1960, p 93). As a nurse, the researcher is able to establish a relationship with both patients and nurses which will not only preserve the humanity of the encounter but may also contribute to the success of the research.

The major instrument for the collection of data is the investigator himself. Thus, the successful employment of the method of participant-observation is predicated by one's ability to establish rapport and relationships of mutual trust and respect with his informants. (Ragucci, 1972, p 487)

Initially, there may be some uncertainty in the mind of a researcher concerning the issues of objectivity and bias arising from the participant-observer role combined with the role as nurse. Such inner uncertainty may be fuelled by comments from others who, according to Agar, will seek to understand the research in the light of the traditional quantitative perspective by asking such questions as: 'What's your hypothesis?' 'What's the independent variable?' 'How can you generalise with such a small sample?' (Agar 1986, p 70). Zigarmi and Zigarmi agree that this can be a real cause for concern to the researcher who is seeking to use the processes of discovery to attach meaning to the activities occurring within a particular social setting, such as nursing.

> The pressure the ethnographer experiences to do good, credible research, is felt throughout the time it takes to do the study . . . In part, the dilemma the ethnographer experiences stems from wanting to do a credible, significant study, yet doubting his/her ability to contend with the constraints and limitations of a qualitative research methodology and to cope with problems related to bias, influence and sampling. (Zigarmi and Zigarmi, 1979, p 32)

However, Lofland offers a word of advice on this issue: '. . . in doing a qualitative study, do not try frontally to play the quantitative game. The games are different' (Lofland, 1971, p 62). Not only is the researcher who uses a qualitative method acting according to a different set of rules, but the field role of 'observer as participant' gives the researcher increased opportunities for gaining insights and attaching meaning to events.

> Because the researcher is involved, a range of modes of awareness can be used in data collection. Empathic and intuitive awareness, for example, are deliberately and purposefully employed. (Oiler, 1982, p 179)

The research problem as stated − What is happening here? − required a methodology that would permit examination of the complexity of nursing in action in its natural setting. Having explored the issues associated with the conduct of qualitative research as a nurse reseacher and accepting the appropriateness of this approach for this study, the next step was to identify the particular methodology to be used in the study.

The Grounded Theory Method

Glaser and Strauss formulated their methodology for the discovery of theory from the systematic collection and analysis of data in 1967. The method arose from their own experiences doing fieldwork among dying people. In the intervening years a literature has developed in amplification and support of the method. Some of this is used to support the following introduction to the grounded theory approach.

Grounded theory 'has rules and procedures which, if carefully followed, produce an analysis of a social context which has both accuracy and applicability' (Stern, 1980, p 23). This discussion will focus on these 'rules and procedures' − as they have been developed by Glaser and Strauss. However, the originators of the method are sure that theirs is not the definitive statement. In their major exposition of the method, they state:

> And so we offer this book, which we conceive as a beginning venture in the development of improved methods for discovering grounded theory. (Glaser and Strauss, 1967, p 1)

Glaser confirms this openness to modification and extension of the method in his later work when he recounts the experiences others have had with the method since 1967.

> Others have done more by trying to take grounded theory in a new direction. This latter was a goal of ours in Discovery when we affirmed that the book was for openers, and that others could take the method in any direction they wished. (Glaser, 1978, p 158)

He goes on to identify the common aspirations of non-sociologist researchers who have used the method.

> All had wanted to discover what the problem is, what processes account for its solution and have tried to get away from the preconceiving nature of other methodologies, where hypotheses are derived from literature and then experimented upon, verified and/or surveyed . . . . More and more people wish to discover what is going on, rather than assuming what should be going on, as required in preconceived type research. (ibid, pp 158–9)

The method, as developed to date, had appeal for several reasons. Firstly, the method's strategies have been documented as a step-by-step process that gives the novice considerable assistance during a very complex procedure. Secondly, it supports the researcher seeking to generate theory in a situation where there is a dearth of theory, as in nursing practice. Thirdly, application of the method can be viewed as a liberating experience that gives the researcher freedom to be fully involved in creative research and theory-building guided by a facilitating approach which supports modification and extension of its processes.

Discussion of the research approach has been organised into five sections: Formulation of the Research Problem, Generation of a Grounded Theory, Use of Literature, Criticism of the Method, and Use of the Method in this Study. This discussion is brief; for an in-depth explanation, the reader is referred to Glaser and Strauss (1967) and Glaser (1978).

Formulation of the Research Problem

In the grounded theory approach, the researcher has an identified general area of concern which requires investigation. The goal is to build a theoretical analysis of the data which will at least describe, but may also explain what is happening and even have a predictive quality.

> To date . . . the grounded theory approach has been used primarily to develop rich substantive analyses. A theoretical analysis at the substantive level, though more modest in scope and power than formal theory, gives the analyst tools for explaining his or her data as well as tools for making predictions. (Charmaz, 1983, p 126)

Within the method there is no 'preconceived framework of concepts and hypotheses' to prescribe the specific data for collection (Glaser, 1978, p 44). Rather, the 'grounded theory study is done to produce abstract concepts and propositions about the relationships between them' (Chenitz and Swanson, 1986, p 8). When the researcher is a nurse rather than a sociologist, the problem to be investigated represents an area of professional concern to the researcher in the role of nurse.

This nursing perspective on the problem for investigation is a legitimate extension of the grounded theory method which advocates 'complete openness' to the data (Glaser, 1978, p 158). Stern gives support by asserting that the 'strongest case for the use of grounded theory is in investigations of relatively uncharted waters, or to gain a fresh perspective in a familiar situation' (Stern, 1980, p 20).

Generation of a Grounded Theory

A key aspect of the grounded theory method is the interrelationship between the collection, coding and analysis of data. Theoretical sampling, the label assigned to this complex process, is the

> . . . data collection for generating theory whereby the analyst jointly collects, codes, and analyses his data and decides what data to collect next and where to find them, in order to develop his theory as it emerges. (Glaser and Strauss, 1967, p 45)

During the period preceding entry into the field, the researcher makes initial decisions on the kind of data to be collected. Many kinds of data are considered relevant and such activities as interviewing, observing and reading documents may proceed simultaneously. Concurrent analysis of the early data may lead to decisions to collect additional data using any method appropriate in the setting.

> Different kinds of data give the analyst different views or vantage points from which to understand a category and to develop its properties; these different views we have called slices of data. (ibid, 1967, p 65)

Coding and memoing are two key activities in theoretical sampling, with both commencing as soon as data collection begins. Soon after it has been collected, the field data is analysed line by line in an attempt to understand what is happening.

Two different types of coding are used: substantive and theoretical (Glaser, 1978). Substantive coding attempts to capture in conceptual form the substance of the data gathered from the field. As the data are analysed line by line, the analyst attempts to look at them from every angle. It is a process of breaking the data down into meaningful conceptual units which seem, according to the intuition and insights of the researcher, to explain what is happening in the data. No assumptions are made that any variables are significant until they emerge from the data as meaningful codes. The labels assigned to the codes arise from within the data, and often use the actual words of informants.

Theoretical coding, the second form, refers to the conceptualisation of the relationship between the substantive codes to form an integrated theoretical representation of the data. 'They [theoretical codes], like substantive codes, are emergent; they weave the fractured story back together again' (ibid, p 72). Although several theoretical codes may fit the same data, Glaser advises the analyst, in any one work, to focus on the development of only one integrative pattern – usually a process – to explain what is happening.

> Since the theory must be grounded, verifying its fit and relevance requires patience in going over and over the data to be sure it works with ease, before a secure investment is taken in selective coding for a focus or a core variable. (ibid, p 61)

Memoing is an important activity associated with coding. As the researcher proceeds with the coding activity, paper and/or tape recorder are always nearby in readiness for the immediate recording of ideas.

> Memos are the theorizing write-up of ideas about codes and their relationships as they strike the analyst while coding. Memos lead, naturally, to abstraction or ideation. Memoing is a constant process that begins when first coding data, and continues through reading memos or literature, sorting and writing papers or monograph to the very end. Memo-writing continually captures the 'frontier of the analyst's thinking' as he goes through either his data, codes, sorts and writes . . . . The four basic goals in memoing are to theoretically develop *ideas* (codes), with complete *freedom* into a memo *fund*, that is highly *sortable*. (ibid, p 83)

As the data are closely examined, coded and analysed, any ideas that strike the analyst about the data, codes, relationships, concepts, and experiences within and outside the current research are recorded, separate from the data, and kept for regular referral and sorting. Glaser and Strauss view this process of thinking and reflecting on the data and the categories as they emerge during coding as of fundamental importance because the 'root sources of all significant theorizing are the sensitive insights of the observer himself' (Glaser and Strauss, 1967, p 251). They propose a rule to be followed in the case of a flash of insight: 'Stop coding and record a memo on your ideas' (ibid, p 107).

Collection of data stops when the researcher finds that similar data are being collected over and over again so that there is no further development of the theoretical categories and their properties which are being generated from the data (ibid, p 61). This process, labelled theoretical saturation, indicates that the analysis is yielding a perspective on the data from which a theory can be generated.

> At the beginning, there is more collection than coding and analysis; the balance then gradually changes until near the end when the research involves more analysis, with brief collection and coding for picking up loose ends. (ibid, p 72)

In addition to theoretical sampling, a second concurrent process is essential to the generation of a grounded theory. Glaser and Strauss have called this the constant comparative method (ibid, p 101–115). Each code is compared with the coding of previous similar incidents. Memos are sorted, codes are grouped and, eventually, a core integrating category or social process will emerge which seems to explain the data. As the process of theoretical saturation occurs at the level of the coding, and the properties of the core integrating category or process become stabilised, the grounded theory begins to take shape.

According to the method, the emerging theory is ready for sharing when it 'explains, with the fewest possible concepts, and the greatest possible scope, as much variation as possible in the behaviour and problem under study' (Glaser, 1978, p 125). At this point, the theoretical outcome is tested by sharing it with the subject group.

> The final test of accuracy comes from the subject group. If a theory fits, mouths drop open, eyes light up, and the audience, grasping the idea, fairly shouts its acceptance. 'That's it,' they say, 'that's just the way it is!' Or they may say, 'Oh of course' as in, 'Of course, who doesn't know that'. (Stern, Allen and Moxley, 1984, p 376)

Glaser articulates a similar view but extends the test to a requirement that the people in the area of the study should see the grounded theory as 'useful' because it 'gives traction over action; it makes sense, by making theoretical sense of common sense' (Glaser, 1978, p 14).

Use of Literature in the Grounded Theory Method

Literature has a limited place in the grounded theory approach. Glaser and Strauss argue that a field study may be distorted by the widespread consultation of literature. They emphasise the power of literature in their argument that the library itself can be a rich source of data for the induction of theory.

> When someone stands in the library stacks, he is, metaphorically, surrounded by voices begging to be heard . . . . people converse, announce positions, argue with a range of eloquence, and describe events or scenes in ways entirely comparable to what is seen and heard during field work. (Glaser and Strauss, 1967, p 163)

These powerful voices speaking from literature are viewed with considerable caution. It is argued that an in-depth literature review of the research problem may lead to an intrusion of concepts from the literature and a biased perspective on the collection and analysis of field data that may prove to be a barrier to openness and discovery in the mind of the researcher (Glaser, 1978, pp 31-32). The fear is that rich emergent categories will fail to be recognised and developed in favour of borrowed categories which have a poor and/or limited fit with the data.

> An effective strategy is, at first, literally to ignore the literature of theory and fact on the area under study, in order to assure that the emergence of

categories will not be contaminated by concepts more suited to different areas. (Glaser and Strauss, 1967, p 37)

In her defence of the grounded theory method, Charmaz contends that researchers can use the relevant literature appropriately 'to expand and clarify the codes and to sensitize themselves to ways of exploring the emerging analysis' (Charmaz, 1983, p 117).

It is significant that Glaser and Strauss were primarily advocating the use of their method to sociologists. The tabula rasa ideal cannot be applied to researchers examining their own arena of professional practice. A nurse researcher cannot pretend that there is no background of experience and knowledge, as well as some familiarity with the literature and the nursing setting, to influence the research conduct and outcomes. This role has already been examined and the claim made that this dual role is a viable one that can be exercised in a study using the grounded theory approach. Therefore, the researcher who is a nurse, while always remaining 'grounded' in the field data and using this as the primary source for the emergent theory, will also acknowledge that the study is 'grounded' within current nursing theory and knowledge.

Criticism of the Grounded Theory Method

Glaser and Strauss admit to using 'frank polemic' in their presentation of the strategies of the grounded theory method, which was their response to the prevailing climate of opinion on the development of sociological theory in the 1960s (Glaser and Strauss, 1967, p 259). This enthusiastic advocacy of the method is continued by Glaser (1978) and is present in their other publications (Glaser and Strauss 1968, 1971; Fagerhaugh and Strauss 1977; Strauss and Glaser 1977). Since its inception, the grounded theory method has been subject to criticism, usually by those who espouse another methodological approach. Several examples will be presented together with comments arising from the experience of its use in this study.

Oiler, defending the phenomenological approach, takes grounded theory to task for its assumption that there will be a discoverable process in the data (Oiler, 1983). Similarly, an advocate of the method has identified two potential pitfalls in its use: premature closure and failing to find a core variable to integrate the analysis (Wilson, 1985, p 423). She suggests the former often comes about when time constraints associated with deadlines lead to an end 'to theoretical sampling and coding before the full range and variation for codes and categories have been discovered' (ibid, p 423). The latter leaves the researcher wondering 'how to salvage the study', but a descriptive report is always an option (ibid, p 423). In this study, both 'pitfalls' were experienced, but time, effort, increasing familiarity with the method, and systematic analysis and re-analysis of the data associated with many creative insights, ultimately led to an integrated theoretical outcome. The researcher's experience confirmed the need to clearly understand the method in order to ensure the investigator is not left with 'mountains of data' with no sense of direction (Simms, 1981, p 359).

In a paper dealing with the problem of rigour in qualitative research in nursing, Sandelowski speaks of the potential hazards associated with involvement with activities and personnel in the field that await a nurse as researcher.

> The researcher in qualitative inquiry is more likely to have direct access to a subject's experience, but may also be unable to maintain the distance from those experiences required to describe or interpret them in a meaningful way. (Sandelowski, 1986, p 31)

Each researcher requires considerable wisdom to maintain an appropriate degree of detached closeness, as distinct from total objectivity, in any field study using participant observation. Glaser and Strauss give emphasis to the difficulty in their call for the field researcher to be 'sufficiently immersed in the world to know it', but to have 'retained enough detachment to think theoretically about what he has seen and lived through' (Glaser and Strauss, 1965, p 7). This involvement is clearly carried through into the development of theory which, they contend, emerges from the analyst's perceptions, personal experiences, and 'hard-won analyses' (ibid, p 6). Thus, the generation of theory from field data requires the creative but measured involvement of the researcher through all stages. The grounded theory method openly challenges those who suggest that complete objectivity is possible in any study involving the actions and thinking of a person occupying the role of researcher.

> The root source of all significant theorizing is the sensitive insights of the observer himself . . . . the researcher can get – and cultivate – crucial insights not only through his research (and from his research) but from his own personal experiences prior to or outside it. (Glaser and Strauss, 1967, pp 251–252)
>
> . . . the so-called 'emergence of categories' involves a complex interplay between 'what's going on out there' and 'what's going on inside' the researcher's head. (Fagerhaugh and Strauss 1977, p 311)

While grounded theory is considered to be a qualitative methodology, both qualitative and quantitative data, indeed any data, can be used to develop a grounded theory (Glaser and Strauss, 1967). Thus, the criticism of the data used to generate the theory will primarily be specific to each study rather than to the method itself. However, the grounded theory approach is clearly considered a qualititative approach in the controversy between quantitative and qualitative research strategies.

Graphic criticism of the method comes from Ford who questions the ability of the researcher to capture 'reality' in a grounded theory.

Those RABBITS [scientists] are horribly mistaken who rely upon so-called procedures of induction . . . for the discovery of 'true' theories. These methods can lead no one to discover anything . . . . he has 'discovered' nothing; what he has done is to link observations together in a haphazard way and then invented a FAIRY TALE [connection of ideas in the form of an explanatory story, or theory] to explain them. (Ford, 1975, pp 139–140)

Glaser and Strauss defend the inductive mode of theory generation and counter such criticism by asserting that 'discovery cannot be stopped, but breaks through both verifications and preconceived conceptual schemes' although it is often not developed in such circumstances (Glaser and Strauss, 1967, p 185). Critics are also answered, if not satisfied, by the method's 'final test of accuracy' – the ability of those in the field to identify their reality with the grounded theory emerging from the research process (Stern et al, 1984, p 376).

The qualitative/quantitative controversy has a large literature and cannot be covered adequately in this brief discussion. Nor can attention be given to the related debate on the issues of validity, reliability and bias in field work, participant observation, and case studies. However, the conflicting perspectives are acknowledged and the decision to use a qualitative approach for this study was made with an awareness of the arguments for and against the method. Indeed, interest in using a qualitative approach in general, and the grounded theory approach in particular, was fuelled by the controversy!

Finally, it is necessary to justify the description of the research outcome as a grounded theory in the face of potential criticism. According to its originators, a grounded theory may be either 'discussional' – systematic description of concepts – or 'propositional' – presentation of a set of propositional statements (Glaser and Strauss, 1967, p 115). In both cases they refer to a group of emergent conceptual categories organised within an integrating framework. Glaser and Strauss consider the discussional type is 'often sufficiently useful at the exploratory stage of theory development' but can, if required, be further developed into the propositional form (ibid, p 115). Thus, grounded theories may vary considerably in their degree of development.

This argument in support of the use of the term 'theory' to describe the discussional form will not be convincing for readers who hold a more traditional definition of theory or who have no personal experience with the methodology. Consequently, the description of the Nursing Partnership as a grounded theory will be open to criticism. However, it does meet the criteria for labelling as a grounded theory of the discussional type. Conceptual categories have been generated; a framework which fits the data has been used to integrate the concepts; statements have been made to claim the existence of both the categories and their placement within the overall framework. It is a theory that describes the various elements within the process of giving and receiving nursing. As yet, it lacks propositional statements which posit formal relationships, particularly of cause and effect and prediction.

Consideration of some of the perplexingly confusing nursing literature on theory, conceptual models, theoretical models and frameworks fails to yield a universally acceptable alternative label for the Nursing Partnership (Dickoff, James and Wiedenbach, 1968; National League for Nursing, 1978; Stevens, 1979; Riehl and Roy, 1974; Chinn and Jacobs, 1983; Walker and Avant, 1983; Fawcett, 1984; Meleis, 1985). Following a similar investigation, Meleis decided to 'relegate most of the differences to semantics' and concluded that 'the final choice of label is a personal matter', although the term '"theory" is sufficient to describe the conceptualisations that have been proposed by our theorists' (Meleis, 1985, p 96).

After considerable reflection, the decision was made to acknowledge the terminology of the method – 'grounded theory' – while accepting that the Nursing Partnership is a theory still in the process of development. At this stage it is closely related to a theoretical or conceptual framework when this is defined as a network of interrelated concepts representing an abstraction induced from reality. Support for this interpretation comes from Glaser and Strauss themselves who use the terms 'analytical framework' and 'theoretical framework' in their discussion of an emergent grounded theory (Glaser and Strauss, 1965, p 6). Therefore, using this precedent, the terms 'theoretical framework' or 'conceptual framework' as defined are used synonymously to describe the outcome of this study.

Using the Grounded Theory Method

In retrospect, the method was appropriate for the study and its use was continually challenging, although the experience was prolonged with many moments of frustration approaching despair.

The process of theoretical sampling – concurrent data collection, coding and analysis – was difficult to sustain. Initially all went well. Eventually, a judgement was made that the case studies being collected were showing a sameness that seemed to indicate that little new information was being collected. In addition, the time available for data collection was drawing to a close. When the fieldwork ended, multiple codes had been identified by the process of line-by-line substantive coding, but an integrating concept was not yet evident.

After the conclusion of data collection, the data were worked over and over again during the process of analysis. Connections were sought between events, between subjects, between codes. The search for meaning in the data continued as an interplay between the general and the particular as ideas for integrating a variety of concepts were tested and discarded. Finally, an integrating social process emerged that synthesised the codes into an integrated theoretical interpretation of the data.

Confirmation for the evolving theoretical framework and its constituent concepts was found within the data.

Discovery of this framework required far more time and effort than anticipated. There is no doubt that, 'as with any research methodology, the living process is less orderly than its written description' (Stern, 1980, p 23). The amount of data was extremely large and required the development of a management system to control it. Transcription of the taped field data took many months. Once an integrating category was identified, a re-analysis of the total data was undertaken with the focus now on validating each constituent category within the emerging theoretical framework. Confidence in the grounded theory approach was increased when this process confirmed the fit between the codes and the data.

Finally, as previously stated, the concurrent nursing work of the researcher meant that the reading of nursing literature was maintained throughout the study. During the life of the research there was a continuing interaction between the professional self and the researcher role. Substantive and theoretical codes were reflected upon from a nursing perspective and placed in the context of current nursing theory and practice. As a consequence, the process of theory generation was much more complex and less isolated from external bias than that suggested by Glaser and Strauss. While this may be criticised from a purist methodological perspective, it is necessary for the nurse researcher to have confidence that the theoretical outcome is identifiable as nursing and that it expands current nursing knowledge.

APPENDIX 2
The Research Protocol

The research protocol used in this study has been separated into components and is discussed under the following headings: The Research Problem, The Research Setting, Entry into the Field, The Study Population, The Field Experience, Summary of the Data, Generating the Grounded Theory and Limitations of the Study.

The Research Problem

The problem for examination was expressed as a general question: What is happening here? This open question was in the mind of the researcher as she entered the familiar setting of the surgical ward to observe the giving and receiving of nursing. A number of patients were followed through their experience of receiving nursing while undergoing elective surgery, and their experiences provided data for the grounded theory. From these case studies came a fresh interpretation of nursing in action based on a range of data systematically collected in the field.

The Research Setting

The setting for this study was a regional teaching hospital of about 900 beds situated close to the centre of a city. The five surgical wards which were chosen for data collection were namely three general surgical wards, an ophthalmology ward and a genito-urinary ward (see glossary in Appendix 4).

Both the ophthalmology and genito-urinary wards are situated within a three-storey block opened in 1944. There is a T-shaped corridor from which doors open into one, two and four-bedded rooms. The three general wards are situated in a newer multi-storey block. One, four and six-bedded rooms open into the outside of an m-shaped corridor with the four-bedded room in each ward being used primarily for patients in the immediate postoperative period after major surgery.

During the study, two wards were staffed by a charge nurse heading a team primarily composed of staff nurses with some enrolled nurses. One of these wards was using primary nursing while the other used a combination of cubicle nursing and task assignment (see glossary in Appendix 2).

Three wards were staffed by a charge nurse with a team of staff nurses, enrolled nurses and a small number of hospital-based student nurses. These wards used a combination of cubicle and team nursing. Three of the other wards used in the study had students from the nearby technical institute school of nursing who were on the wards during the study.

Entry into the Field

Before the study began, permission to undertake the study was given by the nursing administration within the hospital and, with their support, the proposal was forwarded to, and approved by, the hospital's Research Ethical Committee.

A date was established for commencing the study in each ward in succession. The study was discussed with the charge nurse and the nursing staff in the ward. Morning and afternoon staff were addressed at a pre-arranged time during the changeover period of 2.30–3.30 pm. Nurses who were not present at that meeting received a personal explanation if they were assigned to nurse a patient in the study. All five charge nurses were interested and enthusiastic about the research. Variable amounts of interest and enthusiasm were shown by other nursing staff, although no overt opposition was encountered at any time.

The last step before making an appointment to meet each patient was to discuss the study with the potential subject's surgeon. No difficulties were encountered in gaining the support of the surgeons, although the qualitative methodology proved a little difficult for them. Indeed, one surgeon even commented that the study seemed to be a case of 'Clayton's research – the research you do when you're not doing research!' This proved to be a real-life reminder of the continuing qualitative-quantitative controversy.

The Study Population

The study population comprised a group of patients undergoing planned surgery and the nurses responsible for their care.

TABLE 33: Criteria for selection of patient participants

On the waiting list for elective surgery
Resident within the local region
Able to speak English adequately enough to respond
    during interviewing
Sixteen years of age or over
Willing to participate in the study

Patients

Patients were chosen from the list of people waiting to be admitted to the five surgical wards.

Consistent with the goal of studying the situational reality of the surgical experience, there were minimal qualifying criteria for participation in the study. These are listed in Table 33.

Twenty-one patients were in the study population. A small number were followed concurrently in each of the five wards in succession: three in each of the first two wards; four, five and six respectively in the remaining wards. Persistent postoperative complications experienced by two patients caused the researcher to spend much more time than anticipated in the second ward. This led to some anxiety as the Christmas period, with its associated closure of waiting list admissions, drew nearer. Consequently, the number of patients followed concurrently was increased. However, in retrospect, it was recognised that three was the optimal number with a methodology which required simultaneous data collection and analysis. Any increase above this number meant that less time was spent with each patient with a consequent reduction in the breadth of data. More time was required for interviewing, leaving less time for participant observation of activities as they occurred. Analysis, in the form of coding and memoing, was fitted in between visits during the day but was primarily an overnight activity.

Selection was consistent with the protocol for 17 of the 21 patients. Admissions scheduled for the first day on which the researcher would enter the ward were considered for inclusion in list order. Only one such person was excluded because of her inability to converse in English. The remaining 17 were willing to participate in the study. In addition, three waiting list admissions who were already in the ward but were also on the operating schedule for the following day were included. All three met the criteria for participation in the study.

In one ward the charge nurse specifically asked if a patient could be included in the study. She was concerned about this man and was seeking assistance from the researcher, as nurse. Although admitted urgently for observation the previous week, he was scheduled for surgery on the same day as the waiting list patients in the study. In the face of this specific request, this patient was included. Consideration was given to excluding the data on this patient from the analysis, but the flexibility of the research approach permits such situational amendments to the protocol to be made. So, these data were retained.

The study was fully explained to each patient and questions were answered prior to agreement to participate being obtained in writing. A copy of the consent form is included as Appendix 5. No attempt was made to conceal the nature and purpose of the research. Confidentiality of name

TABLE 34: Characteristics of the patient group

Total No:	21		
Sex:	15 Men		
	6 Women		
Marital Status:	15 Married/Partners		
	3 Single		
	2 Widowed		
	1 Divorced		
Age:		Men	Women
	Under 20	0	1
	20–39	2	1
	40–59	6	1
	60–79	7	3
Occupation:	Cafeteria Assistant		Chef
	Clerk (r)		Clerk – Executive
	Clerk – Supervisor		Housewife
	Housewife (r)		Journalist
	Managing Director (r)		Marketing Manager
	Minister's Wife (r)		Office Manager
	Painter/Paperhanger (r)		Personnel Officer
	Plumber		Policeman (r)
	Real Estate Salesman		Sales Manager
	Shoemaker (r)		Shop Assistant (r)
	Storeman (r)		
(r) = retired			

was assured and patients knew that their experiences would be included as part of a dissertation. Although an astute reader could discover the name of the institution, the wards and the dates of the study, and individual anecdotes are used to illustrate the theoretical presentation, and maximum anonymity has been preserved. The total experience of each patient has been merged in the analysis of the field data.

Table 34 summarises the characteristics of the patient group.

The proportion of men was unexpected, but reflects the situation at the time of the study. Similarly, it was surprising that all the patients were Pakeha (of European descent). The age range for both men and women was large although only four were under 40 years of age.

Table 35 lists the types of surgery experienced by the patients in the study. The number of similar operations performed during the period of

TABLE 35: Types of surgery included in the study

	In Study	Total
Block dissection of lymph nodes	1	3
Blocked gortex graft	1	3
Bowel resection	1	20
Carotid endartarectomy	2	14
Cataract extraction	1	57
Gastrectomy	2	7
Inguinal herniorrhaphy	1	27
Injection of oesophageal varices		7
Keratoplasty	1	2
Mastectomy	2	12
Parathyroidectomy	1	3
Sphincterotomy	2	9
Thyroidectomy	1	6
Trabeculectomy	1	8
Transurethral resection	2	26
Ureteroplasty	1	1

data collection is also included. This number is listed alongside each operation.

Fifteen of the patients entered hospital the day before surgery; two were admitted two days before; and four spent four to six days in the ward prior to surgery. The time spent in hospital after surgery varied from two to 20 days. Ten had been discharged by the fifth day, another six had gone home within 10 days and only one was hospitalised for more than 15 days.

Nurses

Individual nurses participated in the study in one or more of three ways according to the nature of their association with the patients in the study. Firstly, at the end of each nursing shift the nurse who was identified as being primarily responsible for nursing the patient during the past eight hours was interviewed. Eighty-two different nurses were interviewed during the study. The five charge nurses were also interviewed. Some baseline data on the nurses who were interviewed were collected and are summarised in Table 36.

Secondly, copies were made of all nursing records maintained on each patient subject while in hospital. The primary records were the nursing history, nursing notes, and nursing care plan. Finally, some nurses participated in the study by their involvement in incidents of interaction

TABLE 36: Charactertistics of the nurse group

Total No:	87	
Status:	5	Charge nurses
	55	Staff nurses
	5	Enrolled nurses
	22	Students
Working hours:	68	Full-time
	19	Part-time
Registration of qualified staff:	3	General nurses
	45	General/obstetric nurses
	12	Comprehensive nurses
	5	Enrolled nurses
Training school of qualified staff:	34	Local hospital boards
	6	Local technical institutes
	14	Other NZ hospital boards
	6	Other technical institutes
	5	Overseas
Students	20	General/obstetric programme
	2	Comprehensive programme

between patient and nurse, and social interaction between nurses in the presence of the researcher. These were recorded as field notes.

The Field Experience

For data collection purposes, the patient's surgical experience was divided into three stages: Stage 1 – Before Admission to Hospital, Stage 2 – The Period of Hospitalisation, and Stage 3 – After Discharge from Hospital. The protocol for each stage will be briefly discussed.

Stage 1 – Before Admission to Hospital

In the protocol, a home visit prior to admission was planned for each patient. This visit had three purposes. Firstly, the researcher would explain the study and ensure the person understood what was required before inviting them to complete the consent form. Secondly, the relationship between researcher and subject would be initiated prior to the stress of admission to the hospital. Thirdly, data collection would commence at this time using three methods: Interview, Observation, and Diary.

Interview: This was planned to be an open-ended but focused conversation between the researcher and the patient which would be recorded. A copy of the interview protocol is presented in Appendix 4. Each interview was to start with an initiating question, and issues would be explored as they arose during the conversation. At all times the researcher attempted to remain sensitive to the person's willingness and ability to discuss each topic.

The first interview was planned to collect data on the person's perception of the world. It was anticipated that the conversation would naturally lead – at an early or late stage – to a discussion on the person's health status and history including the forthcoming surgery.

Observation: During the visit, the researcher planned to note the environment in which the person lived, the person's physical appearance and verbal/non-verbal behaviour patterns. The guide for these observations is presented in Appendix 3.

Diary: At the conclusion of this first visit, participants were to be given a notebook in which they were invited to keep a diary from then until the final visit after discharge from hospital. The patients would be requested to record anything concerning the upcoming experience that they would like to share with the researcher.

Despite this plan, the first experience with Stage 1 visits precipitated a major change in the protocol. Dynamic changes occur in patient loads within individual wards, and the anticipated lead time between notification and admission did not prove to be reality. In the first ward, the researcher obtained the names of three anticipated admissions two days prior to the event. One could not be contacted, one was willing to receive a home visit and one felt it would be better, for the researcher, if the visit were to take place at his workplace. These two visits, hastily arranged for the day before admission, and an event on the day of admission, led to a change in protocol. This experience is recounted in order to explain the circumstances that led to the change.

On arriving for the home visit, the door was opened by a charming elderly man – the patient – who immediately, while leading the way into his lounge, commenced to share personal information relevant to the study. With the tape recorder still in her bag and the consent still unsigned, the researcher was graciously entertained with afternoon tea and social conversation intermingled with the desired interview information. Almost every topic the researcher had anticipated covering during a spontaneous recorded interview was covered. Finally, after completion of the formalities relating to the explanation of the research and the signing of the consent form, the tape recorder was prepared for use. At this point, the man picked up the recorder, took some time to prepare what he wanted to say and gave a six-minute 'speech' in which he recalled the events leading up to the need for the surgery. The visit lasted nearly two hours; the actual recording lasted only six minutes and lacked spontaneity.

Later that day a visit was made to the place of work of the second patient. Although this man continually gave the assurance that all was well, work colleagues kept on entering his office for advice. In this setting the researcher felt intrusive and uncomfortable. The resulting conversation was affected by the circumstances in which it took place.

On the next day, when these two men were admitted to hospital, the researcher consulted the charge nurse concerning the next waiting list admission. She replied, 'The corneal graft is in. He's being done tomorrow.' With that, she walked out of the office and entered a four-bed cubicle, researcher following behind. On approaching a bed on which a man was sitting reading a magazine, she said, 'This is [   ], she's a nurse and is doing a survey. She would like to speak with you.' At this point, the charge nurse smiled and left the room. This man proved to be the third person from the original list with whom contact had not been possible prior to admission. As this was the beginning of the research, and the other Stage 1 interviews had raised unexpected problems, the researcher decided to try undertaking the first interview on admission. The researcher's diary note records: 'I was so pleased I did because I had an excellent conversation with him.'

Thereafter, the Stage 1 interviews were carried out in the hospital as soon as possible after admission. In this environment the preliminaries were soon completed and recording the interview was quickly underway. The initiating questions opened up the conversation and permitted the patients an opportunity to shape their own individual responses. Some immediately spoke of issues relating to the surgery, others started with an account of their childhood. The observation schedule was completed after each Stage 1 interview. Diaries were given to the first three subjects but were not used. Patients reported that they saved up any comments until the researcher's next visit. Thereafter, diaries were given to subjects at the time of discharge but only one entry was made.

Stage 2 – The Period of Hospitalisation

As the focus of the study was on the actual experience of hospitalisation, most data were collected during this second stage in the form of: Patient Interviews, Nurse Interviews, Patient Observation, Nursing Documentation, and Participant Observation.

Patient Interviews: Each patient was to be interviewed three times a day, at the end of the nursing duties at 7 am and 3 pm and the settling of the ward at 9 pm. During each visit a focused conversation was recorded. The tape recorder was small and had a built-in microphone. It was placed on the bed during the interview. Although most patients initially seemed a little uneasy with the recorder, this was much less evident in later interviews.

During each interview, patients were invited to speak of their perceptions of, and reactions to, their current situation and the events of the previous eight hours. A protocol was prepared for the interview and this is presented in Appendix 4. As planned, the exact wording of the initiating question was determined by the circumstances and the patient's status. Most commonly, the conversation commenced with the planned question: 'How have you been since I saw you last?' Although the interviewer guided the duration and scope of each interview, the major determinant was the patient's condition. There were occasions, mostly in the immediate postoperative period, when it was not possible to interview the patient.

Thrice-daily visits were maintained throughout the hospitalisation of the first two patients. At the time of their discharge, the remaining patient in that group was independent and waiting to be discharged in a few days so the visits were reduced to once daily in mid-afternoon. By this stage the researcher was finding the fieldwork, with concurrent transcription and analysis, extremely exhausting. Six to nine hours a day in the ward, divided between three visits, together with the concurrent coding and analysis associated with the research method, had a cumulative effect. It became evident that the planned protocol could not be maintained throughout the months available for the fieldwork. Consequently, the pattern of daily visits was revised. Three visits daily were made during the immediate perioperative period and then the number was reduced to two and, in some cases one, as the patient's condition stabilised and change was less dynamic. The mid-afternoon interview was retained throughout the patient's time in hospital.

Nurse Interviews: Nurse interviews were timed to coincide with patient interviews. The nurse identified as being primarily responsible for nursing the patient during the past duty was interviewed. Each conversation was recorded and commenced with the question: 'Can you tell me about [ ] and the nursing care he(she) has required this duty?' This question sought to ascertain the nurse's perception of her role, the nursing care given during the preceding eight-hour period, and the status of the person at the end of the duty. A copy of the protocol is presented in Appendix 5.

Originally, the intention was to interview only registered nurses. However, in the second ward a number of nurse students were encountered. It transpired that the care of a patient could be assigned to a student who was only nominally under the supervision and guidance of a registered nurse. Therefore, at the end of the duty, the nurse student was identified as the person 'responsible' for the patient during the duty. The protocol was changed to allow interviews with students in such circumstances.

Early in the study, it became apparent that the climate set by the charge nurse could be an important factor in the nursing care offered to patients. This was particularly evident in the variations in the format used for nursing documentation in each ward. Therefore, it was decided to include an interview with the charge nurse towards the end of the data-gathering in each ward.

Observation: During each visit to the patient, the researcher was sensitive to the general condition of the person and their behaviour. The schedule included as Appendix 5 was used to guide these observations.

Nursing Documentation: Duplicate records of the nursing documentation on each patient – nursing notes, nursing history and nursing care plan – were made. In addition, a record of the patient's pain medication and sedation was maintained as this became an important topic in the interviews with nurse and patients. Copies of the two nursing history formats in use are presented in Appendix 6; the two nursing care plan formats are presented in Appendix 7.

Participant Observation: In the field, the researcher wore a uniform with nursing insignia to identify her as a nurse. Her data-gathering activities were acknowledged at all times, as was her status as nurse. As discussed in Appendix 1, she primarily occupied the field role of observer as participant.

During the fieldwork, the researcher participated in informal inter-action with the nursing staff. Comments on the nursing of the patients in the study were noted. Notes were also made of visits made to the patient by nursing and medical staff while the researcher was present.

Planned events involving the patient and a nurse, such as pre-operative teaching or a procedure such as wound care, were included in the study by agreement with the nurse and the patient concerned. It was not possible to observe exactly the same critical events for each patient because several patients were followed at a time and there was consider-able variation between patients. Participation in planned nursing pro-cedures proved to be more difficult than anticipated. A decision was made to collect specific data on the quantity of nursing contact. The total nursing activity involving two patients over a seven-hour period was observed. This confirmed the impression that nursing contact time was considerably less than had been assumed in planning the protocol.

One hundred and twenty-eight incidents directly relevant to the nursing of the subjects were recorded and considered in the analysis.

Instances arose where participation as nurse was appropriate. Such interventions were limited as far as possible, but included verbal assur-ance, counselling, information giving, and activities to maintain safety and patient comfort. These primarily occurred during recorded interviews. Activities of this kind were noted and considered as data, as well as being notified to the patient's nurse if the nurse researcher considered this was appropriate.

Stage 3 – After Discharge from Hospital

Following discharge – at a convenient time for the patient – a final interview took place in the person's home. Once again, this interview took the form of an open-ended but focused discussion between the researcher and the patient subject. It included discussion of the person's memories of the surgery, the hospitalisation and the nursing they received as well as their perception of their present health status. During this visit, it was necessary to end the relationship with the person and allow them to ask questions about any aspects of the research with which they were concerned. A copy of the interview protocol is presented in Appendix 8.

One patient required two home visits. On the first, this elderly man, who had already been readmitted because of a postoperative haemorrhage, was again in considerable distress caused by severe pain and bleeding. Soon after that visit further surgery was required to remedy the problem. A repeat visit was made after his return home. Another patient had already been readmitted to hospital at the time of the Stage 3 visit and, as her life-threatening illness was progressing and the future was uncertain, the interview was recorded in hospital. One patient requested that the interview be held while he underwent renal dialysis in the hospital outpatient unit.

Summary of the Data

The data – from written records, field notes and interviews – are summarised on Table 37.

Generating the Grounded Theory

On the third day of data collection, the field diary contained the following entry:

> Analysis is starting! Thinking about a behavioural category of CONFORMITY – RETENTION OF CONTROL – SELECTIVE CONFORMITY based on . . . .

A multitude of substantive and theoretical codes were recorded and explored. Continuous memoing occurred from the outset. The data were worked in a variety of ways including:

- Line-by-line coding and memoing of all data
- Comparison of content and coding of each type of data in each stage across the patient group

TABLE 37: Summary of data			
Population:	Patients	21	
	Nurses	87	
Interviews:	Stage 1	19	In hospital
		1	At home
		1	At work
	Stage 2	288	Patient
		285	Nurse
	Stage 3	20	At home
		1	In hospital
		1	In outpatient unit
	Charge Nurses	5	
Documentation on each patient (if used):	Nursing notes		
	Nursing care plan(s)		
	Nursing history		
	Medication record		
	Observation record		
	Fluid balance chart		
	Nursing referral to district nurse		
	Medical discharge summary		
Incidents:	128 recorded in field notes		

- Comparison of content and coding of each type of data within each case study
- Memoing on each substantive and theoretical code with reference to the data
- Sorting of the memos and further memoing as codes were grouped and sorted in a variety of ways
- Reduction of the codes into more abstract concepts confirmed by links to data
- Organisation of concepts within an integrative framework followed by a line-by-line recoding of the data in relation to the emergent theory.

By a process of synthesis, the myriad of substantive codes were gradually reduced and developed into fewer concepts with a greater degree of abstraction, although their links to the data were maintained. As this analytical work of discovering meaning continued, there was a search for an integrating framework – a core category or process – to link the concepts into an interpretation that fitted the field situation from which the data were obtained.

Some six months after the completion of data collection, the following diary note was made:

> I had a 'eureka' experience tonight at about 6.40 pm. Believe it or not, I was lying reading in the bath! It was a little too cold to go running down the streets, but the joy in my heart brought tears of gratitude and almost bewilderment to my eyes. What was the 'eureka'? Well, I was reading Glaser and Strauss' 'Status Passage' and, in fact, was only on page 3 when I suddenly realised this was my focus. I am interested in the Nursed Passage, that is, the patient's experience of needing and receiving nursing.

Initially, an attempt was made to apply Glaser and Strauss' theory of Status Passage to the substantive data collected from the field (Glaser and Strauss, 1971). However, the fit between that specific theoretical interpretation of passage and the data was not a comfortable one. Instead, the anthropological concept of passage, as originally proposed by van Gennep, was adapted and extended to provide an integrating framework for the experience of a person undergoing surgery as it was emerging from the data (van Gennep, 1960).

The specific properties of the Nursing Partnership arise from the nursing setting rather than being imposed from the literature. Glaser and Strauss' suggestion that researchers explore for multiple properties characteristic of the particular passage being described, rather than focusing on a single or few derived properties and perhaps neglecting significant data, was followed (Glaser and Strauss, 1971, pp 1–11).

The study led to the emergence of a grounded theory in the 'discussional' form (Glaser and Strauss, 1967, p 115). It is a research-induced theoretical or conceptual framework. At this point, the theory of the Nursing Partnership requires further development before it can be stated in the propositional form.

The challenge facing the researcher was to write the theoretical outcome in a way that would persuade practitioners that it could be relevant to their practice; that the time required to understand it would be worthwhile; and that there would be personal and professional rewards in its use. With this in mind, care was taken to use terminology which is readily understandable by the practising nurse. Indeed, one of the key tests for a grounded theory is the degree to which people in the field can relate it to the reality of their everyday world. Thus it has to be presented in a form which 'makes its fit and relevance easy to comprehend' (Glaser and Strauss 1967, p 32). This is achieved through the use of descriptive terms for the concepts and also by means of the constant use of anecdotes to illustrate the direct link between the theoretical outcome and the reality of nursing as revealed in the data.

Limitations of the Study

Some important limitations are recognised in this study and its outcome. These are primarily consequences of decisions made by the researcher during the development of the research protocol, while in the field and during data analysis.

Data were collected in five surgical wards within one hospital, so there are limitations on how generally the result can be applied. This is consistent with a grounded theory at the stage of development reached in this study. However, the concepts have been developed to a degree of abstraction that potentially lifts them beyond this single setting. Confirmation of the general applicability of the process would come through specific testing of each concept within the framework. The potential for this expansion has been confirmed by the reactions of colleagues to the Nursing Partnership.

Because of the duration of the study and changes in patients and nursing staff, it was not possible to share the emerging theory with the people who provided the data. However, it has been shared along the way with nursing colleagues and students as well as other people who had had recent experiences as patients. There have been many confirmatory statements attesting to the validity of the conceptualisation. Nurses have also spoken with enthusiasm of the potential significance of the research. A number have commented that it 'gives new meaning to nursing'.

At the outset, it was hoped that registered nurses would be the sole source of nursing data. That was not to be. Instead, a decision was made to include nursing students when these were assigned to nurse the patients in the study. Supervision was indirect so that the registered nurse with overall responsibility might not have had any contact with the patient during the nursing shift. Examination of the data from senior students and staff nurses did not reveal any appreciable differences in relation to the dimensions identified in the research outcome, certainly none that would negate the findings.

Another limitation, perhaps more in the retrospective perception of the researcher rather than in reality, was the decision to follow more than three patients at a time in the latter part of the fieldwork. This decision created pressure on the researcher and led to some interviews being lost through technical oversights which were caused by the sheer amount of recording being done. It also meant that less time was available for each patient, especially for just being there to observe incidents as they occurred. Despite this, participant observation, particularly of nurses and patients interacting, although planned to be a major source of data, yielded far less than anticipated. Concern over this lack of observed nurse-patient encounters led to the finding that actual nursing time was considerably less, in amount and frequency, than expected. Therefore, the primary data for the theory were the subjective comments by patients and nurses during recorded interviews. However, these, when supplemented by nursing documentation and the incidents which were recorded, provided a rich and valuable database.

As analysis progressed, the emergent theoretical framework became increasingly complex. Concepts produced by reduction of the multiple substantive codes required subconcepts as their range of properties increased; phases were developed; the working partnership evolved; and, finally, the concept of passage was applied to link the various pieces together. As a consequence, a decision had to be made on whether the focus of the outcome would be on breadth – the whole passage – or depth – a concentrated analysis of a limited number of concepts. The decision – the whole passage – was not hard to make because of the need to establish an overall shape to the novel framework which was emerging. However, this resolution did mean that discussion of each of the many concepts generated from a huge mass of data would be, of necessity, somewhat brief. Much remains unsaid. Anecdotal data have been selectively used to provide depth and relevance to the discussion of the findings. They also add a human touch, giving a sense of the very real people, nurses and patients, who lie behind the generalisations. Many treasures remain hidden in the raw data, awaiting further attention to reveal their value in supporting and extending each concept within the theory.

As this is a report of a research study, the findings have rightly been limited to those emerging from the analysis of the data. However, throughout the experience, the researcher, as nurse, has reflected on where the theory might go from here. Constantly, there has been a temptation to say more, make more decisions, expand a concept, all on the basis of personal experience and accumulated nursing wisdom. This inclination has been overcome, albeit with some difficulty, and the research outcome remains immersed in the data from which it originated. Consequently, the nurse researcher is left overflowing with ideas arising from the experience.

These limitations are acknowledged as part of the study, reflecting the reality that is qualitative research in action. Nevertheless, there is little evidence that they detract from the theoretical outcome.

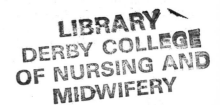

APPENDIX 3
Consent Form to Participate in Study

Area of study: The nursing needs of persons undergoing surgery

Brief description: A number of persons on the waiting list for surgery will be visited before or on admission and interviewed by the researcher. After admission the person will be visited daily and another home visit will be made about one week after discharge. Up to five persons to be admitted to each of a group of surgical wards will be invited to participate in the study

Researcher: Judith C. Christensen, doctoral student, Massey University

Relevant background: Registered nurse with 21 years of experience including 13 years as a teacher and experience as a charge nurse in a surgical ward

Nature of patient involvement in this study:
- An interview before or at time of admission to hospital and after discharge
- Interviews during hospitalisation – short interview at approximately 7 am, 3 pm and 9 pm daily
- Observation – the researcher will make observations of the activities involving the person at various times during the person's stay in hospital

Consent statement:
- I have read the above and have had the opportunity to discuss the study and my part in it with Miss Christensen
- I understand that this study has been approved by the hospital administration and by a special hospital board committee
- I understand that my doctor is aware of my participation in this study
- I know that Miss Christensen will discuss with me any time she wishes to observe activities during my hospital experience, and will seek my permission to do so
- I understand that I may withdraw from this study at any time
- I agree to take part in this study

Signed: _____ Date: _____

APPENDIX 4
Glossary of Nursing and Medical Terms

Charge nurse:	The nurse in charge of a hospital ward
Chronic renal failure:	Progressive loss of kidney function
Corneal graft:	Replacement of a damaged cornea in eye by cornea from a donor
Cubicle nursing:	A system for delivering nursing care by allocating patients to nursing staff according to room or cubicle
Enrolled nurse:	A graduate of a one-year basic nursing programme who works under the supervision of a registered nurse
Gastric ulcer:	An ulcer on the inner wall of the stomach
General surgical ward:	A ward in which a variety of types of surgery are performed
Genito-urinary:	The organs of reproduction together with the organs concerned with production and excretion of urine
Glaucoma:	Group of eye diseases characterised by an increase in pressure within the eye
Haemodialysis:	Removal of toxic wastes from the body through a semipermeable membrane while the blood is circulated outside the body
Hodgkin's disease:	A malignant disease in the lymph nodes, spleen and lymphoid tissue
Hospital-based student:	A nurse student within a school of nursing operated by a hospital board
House surgeon:	A doctor employed by a hospital during the first or second year after medical school
Malignant:	A condition that tends to worsen so as to cause serious illness or death if not treated, as in the case of cancer
Melanoma:	A tumour containing dark pigment that arises from a nevus [mole]
Oesophageal varices:	Varicose veins in the lower gullet caused by liver disease

Ophthalmology:	Area of medicine concerned with the eye
Primary nursing:	A system for delivering nursing care in which patients are assigned to one nurse who plans the nursing and other nurses follow that plan while the primary nurse is off duty
Rectal fissure:	A painful lineal ulcer at the margin of the anus
Registrar:	A doctor three or more years out of medical school employed by a hospital who is undertaking advanced training in a branch of medicine
Renal dialysis:	Same as haemodialysis
Staff nurse:	A registered nurse within a ward nursing team
Task assignment nursing:	A system for delivering nursing care in which nursing work is divided into tasks for distribution among different levels of nursing staff
Technical institute:	A tertiary college within the system of general education
Urinary tract infection:	An infection in the kidneys, bladder, ureter or urethra

APPENDIX 5
Stage 1 Interview Guide and Observation Schedule

Interview Guide

The interview will commence with an initiating question but the conversation will then be determined by the nature of the responses made by the subject and the guiding of the researcher as issues are explored. It is realised that some persons will need more probing and prompting than others. However, it is the researcher's intention to listen and probe appropriately rather than tightly structure the interview.

Primary theme:	The internal and external world of the person
Initiating question:	'I would like to learn something about you and the kind of life you live . . .'
Probes:	Daily pattern of living
	Self
	Self in relation to others
Secondary theme:	Personal health, nature and consequences of change in health status
Initiating question:	'Can you tell me about your own experience of health and illness . . .'
Probes:	Health maintenance activities
	Experience of family health problems
	Attitude to illness and disability
	Present health problem

Observation Schedule

Completed after first interview:

Apparent physical state
Evidence of health problem
Stature and build
Posture and mobility
Dress and grooming
Communication – speech and mannerisms
Manner and mood
Social and physical environment
Other impressions

APPENDIX 6
Stage 2 Interview Guide and
Observation Schedule for Patient

Baseline Data
Time:
Day of hospitalisation:

Interview Guide

The nature of this guided conversation will be determined by the status of the person and his [her] ability to speak. The interview may be very short or may cover a number of issues of current concern to the patient as raised by him [her] in response to the initial question

Theme:	Reflections on past eight hours and own present state
Initiating question:	'How have you been since I saw you last?' or 'How are you feeling now?' or 'Can you tell me what has happened since I saw you last?'
Probes:	Perception of events and own state Feeling about self Sense of control of – self — events Personal concerns Perceived sources of support

Observation Schedule

Description of person – appearance
Equipment in use
Vital signs
Recordings currently in use
Mood and manner during interview
Other significant observations

APPENDIX 7
Stage 2 Interview Guide for Nurse

Baseline data

Date:
Time:
Type of registration:
Year of registration:
Training school:
Time employed − in hospital:
              − in ward:

Interview Guide

Theme:	Nurse's perception of the patient and his/her nursing care
Initiating question:	'Can you tell me about [ ] and the nursing care he/she has required this duty . . .'
Probes:	Patient's status
	Changes during the duty
	Nursing care given to patient
	Individualisation of nursing care
	Information available to nurse
	Relationship with patient
	Perception of nursing
	Anticipatory nursing
	Reactive nursing

APPENDIX 8
Nursing History Forms

General

Patient's Perceptions and Expectations Related to Illness and Hospitalisation
What do you expect is going to happen to you while in hospital?
How long do you expect to be in hospital?
Has your illness affected your lifestyle?
If yes, in what way?

Mobility
Independent
Dependent – Walking stick
          – Walking frame
          – Wheelchair
          – Other

Hygiene
Bath or Shower – Morning or Evening
               – Independent or Dependent
Oral care   – Brushes own teeth or Dependent
               – Dentures
Dressing   – Independent or Dependent
How often do you usually wash your hair?

Rest and Sleep
What time do you normally retire to bed?
Do you have trouble going to sleep or staying asleep?
Do you have anything to help you sleep?
How many pillows do you like?
Do you like ventilation at night?

Elimination

Bladder — Continent or Incontinent
       — Frequency
Bowels — Do you take a laxative? Regularly
                                    Occasionally
                                    Frequently
                                    Never

Communication

Eyes: Do you wear spectacles? Yes or No
           If yes, why?
           If appropriate, what way does your limited eyesight
           handicap you?
Hearing: Do you have any difficulty in hearing? Yes or No
           If yes, do you wear a hearing aid?

Nutrition

What fluids do you prefer to drink?
Do you have any food or fluid dislikes?
Are you on a special diet? Yes or No
If yes, what kind?
Do you have any problems with your diet? Yes or No
Does the condition of your teeth or mouth limit your eating?

Social Needs

Do you live alone? Yes or No
What is your home situation?
Will your relatives/friends be able to visit you? Yes or No
Will you have help from your relatives/friends on discharge? Yes
or No
Would you like the hospital chaplain to visit you? Yes or No
If yes, what denomination?
Has any member of the health services been attending you or any
member of the household? Yes or No
District nurse or public health nurse or social worker or other
(specify)

Nurse's Observations During Interview

Hygiene: Skin condition
          Nails
          Chiropody — Yes or No

Communication Patterns

Quiet
Talkative
Anxious
Depressed
Comfortable
Cooperative
Confused

Summary of Main Points

Surgical

Diagnosis

Previous Hospital Admissions

(Take from medical notes and keep it brief)

Do you remember anything particular about your stay?

Patient's Expectations of Hospital Stay

Why have you come to hospital?
What is your health normally like?
Has anyone explained your surgery/tests to you?
What do you understand by their explanation?
How long do you think you will be in hospital?

Activities of Daily Living

PAIN
Have you any pain?
Describe

SLEEP
Hours of sleep per night
Do you need to get up at night?
If unable to sleep, what do you do?

HYGIENE
Do you have dentures?
Are they in good condition?

CONTINENCE
What are your usual bowel habits?
Do you have bowel irregularities?
What do you take at home for this?
Usual bladder habits
Do you have any trouble with your water?

FEEDING
Were you on a special diet?
Any problems?

AMBULATION
Do you use walking aids?
Do you have difficulty with seeing and hearing?

Assessment of Capabilities

Name of NOK [next of kin]
Do you mind my discussing your condition and progress with him/her?
Has your being admitted made any difference to his/her life?
If alone, are you worried about pets, cancelling orders, rent, etc.
Do you do your own shopping or housework?

Community Care

List community services received prior to admission

Summary

Further Comments

APPENDIX 9
Nursing Care Plan (Surgical)

Name _____

Consultant _____

Birth Date _____ Age _____ Sex _____

Patient No. _____ Ward _____

Diagnosis _____

Date	Nursing Problems	Nursing Aims	Date Resolved
(17 lines)			

Activity Date	Nursing Orders	Signature
Mental State	*(7 lines)*	
Nutrition	*(11 lines)*	
Observations	*(8 lines)*	
Hygiene	*(5 lines)*	
Mobility	*(7 lines)*	
Elimination	*(2 lines)*	
Special Cares	*(22 lines)*	

APPENDIX 10
Stage 3 Interview Guide and Observation Schedule

Baseline Data

Date:
Time:
Place:

Interview Guide

This final interview will be very unstructured, with a free exploration of issues as they arise. Additional questions will be formulated according to patient responses.

Initiating Question: 'I wonder if you could look back and comment on this experience . . .'

Probes: Nurses
Nursing care
Hospitalisation
Present status
Value of surgery
Fulfilment of expectations
Influence of surgery on life
Satisfaction

Observation Schedule

Apparent physical state – appearance
Evidence of recent surgery
Posture and mobility
Dress and grooming
Communication – speech and mannerisms
Manner and mood
Other significant observations

REFERENCES

Agar, M.H. (1986) *Speaking of ethnography*. Beverley Hills, California: Sage Publications.

American Nurses' Association. (1973) *Standards of nursing practice*. Kansas City: American Nurses' Association.

Ashley, J.A. (1976) *Hospitals, paternalism and the role of the nurse*. New York: Teachers College Press.

Benner, P. (1984) *From novice to expert*. Menlo Park, California: Addison-Wesley Publishing Company.

Berry, A.J. and Metcalf, C.L. (1986) Paradigms and practices: the organisation of the delivery of nursing care. *Journal of Advanced Nursing*, 11, 589–597.

Board of Health. (1974) *An improved system of nursing services for New Zealand*. Report Series No. 23. Wellington: Government Printer.

Buckenham, June E. and McGrath, Gerry. *The Social Reality of Nursing*. Sydney: ADIS Health Science Press, 1983.

Burgess, M.E. (1972) The qualified nurse. *New Zealand Nursing Journal*, November, 5.

Byerly, E.L. (1976) The nurse-researcher as participant observer in a nursing setting. In *Transcultural nursing: a book of readings*. Edited by P.J. Brink. Engelwood Cliffs, New Jersey: Prentice-Hall, 143–162.

Carpenter, H. (1971) *An improved system of nursing education for New Zealand*. Wellington: Department of Health.

Carrieri, V.K. and Sitzman, J. (1971) Components of the nursing process. *Nursing Clinics of North America*, 6, 115–124.

Cartwright, S. (1988) *The report of the committee of inquiry into allegations concerning the treatment of cervical cancer at National Women's Hospital and into other related matters*. Auckland: Government Printing Office.

Charmaz, K. (1983) The grounded theory method: an explication and interpretation. In *Contemporary field research*. Edited by R.M. Emerson. Boston: Little, Brown and Company, 109–126.

Chenitz, W.C. and Swanson, J.M. (1986) *From practice to grounded theory*. Menlo Park, California: Addison-Wesley Publishing Company.

Chick, N. (1983) Renaissance or reformation: options for nursing. *Papers presented at Norman Peryer Forum 18–20 November, 1983.* NERF Studies in Nursing: No. 11. Wellington: Nursing Education and Research Foundation.

Chick, N. and Meleis, A.F. (1986) Transitions: A nursing concern. In *Nursing research methodology: issues and implementation.* Edited by P.L. Chinn. Rockville, Maryland: Aspen Systems Corporation, 237–257.

Chinn, P.L. and Jacobs, M.K. (1983) *Theory and nursing.* St. Louis: The C.V. Mosby Company.

Christensen, J.C. (1971) *The impact of a religious education on the moral development of children.* Unpublished research paper.

Christensen, J.C. (1972) *Saline abortion: a study of female behaviour in a crisis situation.* Unpublished research paper.

Christensen, J.C. (1976) After three years. *New Zealand Nursing Journal,* March, 23–24.

Collins English Dictionary. Australian Edition. (1979) Sydney: Collins.

Congalton, A.A. and Najman, J.M. (1971) *Nurse and patient.* Sydney: F.S. Symes Pty Limited.

Coser, R.L. (1962) *Life in the ward.* Michigan: Michigan State University Press.

Department of Education. (1972) *Nursing education in New Zealand.* Report of a committee set up to consider and report to the Minister of Education on recommendation 1.6 of the report of Dr Helen Carpenter entitled 'An improved system of nursing education for New Zealand.' Wellington: Department of Education.

Department of Health. (1969) *A review of hospital and related services in New Zealand.* Wellington: Department of Health.

Deutscher, I. (1975) Foreword to *Introduction to qualitative research methods,* by R. Bogdan and S.T. Taylor. New York: John Wiley & Sons.

Dickoff, J.; James, P. and Wiedenbach, E. (1968) Theory in a practice discipline – part 1: practice oriented theory. *Nursing Research,* 17:5, 415–435.

Fagerhaugh, S.Y. and Strauss, A. (1977) *Politics of pain management: staff-patient interaction.* Menlo Park, California: Addison-Wesley Publishing Company.

Fawcett, J. (1984) *Analysis and evaluation of conceptual models of nursing.* Philadelphia: F.A. Davis Company.

Ford, J. (1975) *Paradigms and fairy tales.* London: Routledge & Kegan Paul.

Gardner,D.L. (1985) Presence. In *Nursing interventions.* Edited by G.M. Bulechek and J.C. McCloskey. Philadelphia: W.B. Saunders Company, 316–324.

Glaser,B.G. (1978) *Theoretical sensitivity*. Mill Valley, California: The Sociology Press.

Glaser, B.G. and Strauss, A.L. (1965) The discovery of substantive theory: a basic strategy underlying qualitative research. *The American Behavioral Scientist*, 8:6, 5–12.

Glaser, B.G. and Strauss, A.L. (1967) *The discovery of grounded theory*. Chicago: Aldine Publishing Company.

Glaser, B.G. and Strauss, A.L. (1968) *Time for dying*. Chicago: Aldine Publishing Company.

Glaser, B.G. and Strauss, A.L. (1971) *Status passage*. Chicago: Aldine Atherton.

Gots, R. and Kaufman, A. (1978) *The people's hospital book*. New York: Crown Publishers, Inc.

Greene, J.A. (1979) Science, nursing and nursing science: a conceptual analysis. *Advances In Nursing Science*, October, 57–64.

Gruendemann, B. J.; Casterton, S.B.; Hesterly, S.C.; Minckley, B.B.; and Shetler, M.G. (1973) *The surgical patient: behavioural concepts for the operating room nurse*. Saint Louis: The C.V. Mosby Company.

Hampton, A. Educational standards for nurses (1894). In King, M.G. Nursing shortage (c. 1915). *Images*, 21:3, 1989, 124–127.

Hansen, M. (1979) Address to 2nd Annual Symposium of Robert Wood Johnson Nurse Faculty Fellowships Program in Primary Care presented April 21 in Nashville, Tennessee.

Henderson, V. (1966) *The nature of nursing*. New York: The Macmillan Company.

Hill, R.J. (1970) On the relevance of methodology. In *Sociological methods*. Edited by N.K. Denzin. Chicago: Aldine Publishing Company, 12–19.

Hinds, P.S. (1984) Inducing a definition of 'hope' through the use of grounded theory. *Journal of Advanced Nursing*, 9, 357–362.

Hoff, L.E. (1978) *People in crisis: understanding and helping*. Menlo Park, California: Addison-Wesley Publishing Company.

Johnson, D. (1968) *One conceptual model of nursing*. Unpublished paper presented April 25 at Vanderbilt University, Nashville, Tennessee.

Johnson, D. (1972) Cardiovascular care in the first person. *ANA Clinical Sessions 1972*. New York: Appleton-Century-Crofts, 127–134.

Johnson, J.E. (1984) Coping with elective surgery. *Annual Review of Nursing Research*, 2, 107–132.

Junker, B.H. (1960) *Field work: an introduction to the social sciences*. Chicago: The University of Chicago Press.

Kaperick, D.P. (1971) The nurse – as a people helper. *New Zealand Nursing Journal*, April, 23.

Kim, H.S. (1983a) *The nature of theoretical thinking in nursing.* Norwalk, Connecticut: Appleton-Century-Crofts.

Kim, H.S. (1983b) Collaborative decision making in nursing: a theoretical framework. In *Advances in nursing theory development.* Edited by P.L. Chinn. Rockville, Maryland: Aspen Systems Corporation, 271–283.

Kim, H.S. (1987) *Collaborative decision making with clients.* Tape of address to International Nursing Conference on Clinical Judgement and Decision Making, Calgary.

King, I.M. (1971) *Toward a theory of nursing.* New York: John Wiley & Sons.

King, I.M. (1978) *Nursing theory.* Tape of address to Second Nurse Educators' Conference, New York.

Kitson, A.L. (1987) Raising standards of clinical practice – the fundamental issue of effective nursing practice. *Journal of Advanced Nursing*, 12, 321–329.

Leininger, M. (1970) *Nursing and anthropology: two worlds to blend.* New York: John Wiley & Sons.

Leininger, M. (1985) Preface to *Qualitative research methods in nursing.* Edited by M. Leininger. Orlando, Florida: Grune & Stratton.

Levine, M.E. (1967) The four conservation principles of nursing. *Nursing Forum*, 6:1, 45–59.

Levitt, R. (1975) Attitudes of hospital patients. *Nursing Times*, March 27, 497–499.

Lofland, J. (1971) *Analysing social settings: a guide to qualitative observation and analysis.* Belmont, California: Wadsworth Publishing Company.

McBride, M.A.; Diers, D.; and Schmidt, R.L. (1970) The nurse-researcher: the crucial hyphen. *American Journal of Nursing*, June, 1256–1260.

McClure, M.L. and Nelson, M.J. (1982) Trends in hospital nursing. In *Nursing in the 1980s: crises, opportunities, challenges.* Edited by L.H. Aiken. Philadelphia: J.B. Lippincott Company, 59–73.

McIntosh, J. and Dingwall, R. (1978) Teamwork in theory and practice. In *Readings in the sociology of nursing.* Edited by R. Dingwall and J. McIntosh. Hampshire, England: Saxon House, 118–134.

MacQueen, J.S. (1974) A phenomenology of nursing. *Nursing Papers*, 6:3, 9–19.

Manthey, M. (1980) *The practice of primary nursing.* Boston: Blackwell Scientific Publications.

Mauksch I.G. and David, M.L. (1974) Prescription for survival. In *The nursing process in practice.* New York: American Journal of Nursing Company, 1–11.

Meleis, A.I. (1985) *Theoretical nursing: development and progress.* Philadelphia: J.B. Lippincott Company.

Miller, A. (1985) The relationship between nursing theory and nursing practice. *Journal of Advanced Nursing*, 10, 417–424.

Mundinger, M.O. (1980) *Autonomy in nursing.* Maryland: Aspen Systems Corporation.

Munhall, P.L. (1982) Nursing philosophy and nursing research: in apposition or opposition? *Nursing Research*, 31:3, 176–178,181.

National League for Nursing. (1978) *Theory development: what, why, how?* New York: National League for Nursing.

New Zealand Nurses' Association. (1973) Nursing education moves. *New Zealand Nursing Journal*, January, 21–23.

New Zealand Nurses' Association. (1976) *New directions in post-basic education.* Wellington: New Zealand Nurses' Association.

New Zealand Nurses' Association. (1980) Changes in nursing education. *New Zealand Nursing Journal*, March, 11–13.

New Zealand Nurses' Association. (1981) *Standards of nursing practice.* Wellington: New Zealand Nurses' Association.

New Zealand Nurses' Association. (1984) *Nursing education in New Zealand: a review and a statement of policy.* Wellington: New Zealand Nurses' Association.

New Zealand Nursing Education and Research Foundation. (1977) *New Zealand nursing manpower planning report.* NERF Studies in Nursing: Number 4. Wellington: Nursing Education and Research Foundation.

Nightingale, A. (1983) Nurses must strive for excellence. *New Zealand Nursing Journal*, October, 22–23.

Nightingale, F. (1859) *Notes on nursing: what it is, and what it is not.* Harrison and Sons; reprint ed., Edinburgh: Churchill Livingstone, 1980.

Oiler, C. (1982) The phenomenological approach in nursing research *Nursing Research*, 31:3, 178–181.

Omery, A. (1983) Phenomenology: a method for nursing research. *Advances in Nursing Science*, January, 49–63.

Orem, D.E. (1971) *Nursing: concepts of practice.* New York: McGraw Hill Book Company.

Orem, D.E. (1978) *Nursing theory.* Tape of address at Second Nurse Educators' Conference, New York.

Orlando, I.J. (1961) *The dynamic nurse-patient relationship.* New York: G.P. Putnam's Sons.

Parker, J. (1985) Cancer passage – the change process in leukaemia. In *Long-term care.* Edited by K. King. Edinburgh: Churchill Livingstone, 96–119.

Parse, R.R. (1981) *Man-living-health: a theory of nursing.* New York: John Wiley & Sons.

Parse, R.R.; Coyne, A.B. and Smith, M.J. (1985) *Nursing research: qualitative methods.* Maryland: Brady Communications Company.

Paterson, J.G. and Zderad, L.T. (1976) *Humanistic nursing.* New York: John Wiley & Sons.

Pearson, A. (Ed.) (1988) *Primary nursing.* London: Croon Helm.

Pearson, A. and Vaughan, B. (1986) *Nursing models for practice.* London: Heinemann Nursing.

Peplau, H.E. (1952) *Interpersonal relations in nursing: a conceptual frame of reference for psychodynamic nursing.* New York: G.P. Putnam's Sons.

Piddington, R. (1952) *An introduction to social anthropology.* Volume One. Edinburgh: Oliver and Boyd.

Pitts, A. (1980) Standards for nursing – their impact on quality care. *New Zealand Nursing Journal,* March, 3–7.

Quint, J.C. (1969) The case for theories generated from empirical data. In *Approaches to nursing research and theory development in nursing.* Proceedings of a symposium held on May 4 1966. New York: American Journal of Nursing, 8–13.

Ragucci, A.T. (1972) The ethnographic approach and nursing research. *Nursing Research,* 21:6, 485–490.

Rangihau, J. (1975) Being Maori. In *Te ao hurihuri.* Edited by Michael King. Wellington: Hicks Smith & Sons Ltd, 221–233.

Remen, N. (1980) *The human patient.* New York: Anchor Press.

Riehl, J.P. and Roy, C. (1974) *Conceptual models for nursing practice.* New York: Appleton-Century-Crofts.

Roberts, K.L. (1980) Nursing: profession or pretender? *The Australian Nurses' Journal,* 9:10, 33–35,51.

Rogers, M. E. (1970) *An introduction to the theoretical basis of nursing.* Philadelphia: F.A. Davis.

Roper, N.; Logan, W.; and Tierney, A. (1980) *The elements of nursing.* Edinburgh: Churchill Livingstone.

Rosenthal, C.J.; Marshall, V.W.; Macpherson, A.S.; and French, S.E. (1980) *Nurses, patients and families.* London: Croon Helm Ltd.

Roy, C. (1976) *Introduction to nursing: an adaptational model.* Englewood Cliffs, New Jersey: Prentice-Hall.

Roy, C. (1984) Framework for classification systems development: progress and issues. In *Classification of nursing diagnoses: proceedings of the Fifth National Conference.* Edited by M.J. Kim; G.K. McFarland; and A.M. McLane. St. Louis: The C.V.Mosby Company, 26–45.

Rubin, R. (1969) A theory of clinical nursing. In *Approaches to nursing research and theory development in nursing.* Proceedings of a symposium held on May 4 1966. New York: American Journal of Nursing, 44–46.

Salmon, E. B. (1982) *A profession in transition*. A Collection of Writings edited by P. Carroll; A. Fieldhouse; and S. Shaw. Wellington: The C.L. Bailey Nursing Education Trust.

Salmond, G.C.; Powell, G.D.; Gray, A.; and Barrington, R. (1977) *A patient opinion survey Wellington Hospital 1974*. Wellington: Department of Health.

Sandelowski, M. (1986) The problem of rigor in qualitative research. *Advances in Nursing Science*, 8:3, 27–37.

Schlotfeldt, R.M. (1972) Approaches to the study of nursing questions and the development of nursing science – introduction. *Nursing Research*, 21:6, 484–485.

Shaw, S.M. (1974) Nursing service without students. *New Zealand Nursing Journal*, April, 3–5,24.

Simmons, L.W. and Henderson, V. (1964) *Nursing research: a survey and assessment*. New York: Appleton-Century-Crofts.

Simms, L.M. (1981) The grounded theory approach in nursing research. *Nursing Research*, 30:6, 256–259.

Smith, D.W. (1981) *Survival of illness*. New York: Springer Publishing Company.

Stein, L.I.; Watts, D.T.; and Howell T. The doctor-nurse game revisited. *New England Journal of Medicine*, 322:8, 546–549.

Stern, P.N. (1980) Grounded theory methodology: its use and processes. *Image*, 12:1, 20–23.

Stern, P.N.; Allen, L.M. and Moxley, P.A. (1984) Qualitative research: the nurse as grounded theorist. *Health Care for Women International*, 5, 371–385.

Stevens, B.J. (1979) *Nursing theory: analysis, application, evaluation*. Boston: Little, Brown and Company.

Strauss, A.L. (1970) *Mirrors and masks: the search for identity*. San Francisco: The Sociology Press.

Strauss, A.L.; Corbin, J.; Fagerhaugh, S.; Glaser, B.G.; Maines, D.; Suczek, B. and Wiener, C.L. (1984) *Chronic illness and the quality of life*. (2nd ed.). St.Louis: The C.V.Mosby Company.

Strauss, A.L. and Glaser, B.G. (1977) *Anguish: a case history of a dying trajectory*. London: Martin Robertson.

Styles, M.M. (1982) *On nursing: toward a new endowment*. St. Louis: The C.V. Mosby Company.

Swanson, J.M. and Chenitz, W.C. (1982) Why qualitative research in nursing? *Nursing Outlook*, April, 241–245.

Tanner, C. (1988) Curriculum revolution: the practice mandate. In *Curriculum revolution: mandate for change*. New York: National League for Nursing, 201–216.

Taylor, C. (1970) *In hospital orbit: hospitals and the cult of efficiency*. New York: Holt, Rinehart and Winston.

Tinkle, M.B. and Beaton, J.L. (1983) Toward a new view of science: implications for nursing research. *Advances in Nursing Science*, January, 27–36.

Toynbee, P. (1977) *Hospital*. London: Hutchinson.

van Gennep, A. (1960) *The rites of passage*. (English translation by S. Kimball). London: Routledge & Kegan Paul.

Walker, L.O. and Avant, K.C. (1983) *Strategies for theory construction in nursing*. Norwalk, Connecticut: Appleton-Century-Crofts.

Watson, J. (1979) *Nursing: the philosophy and science of caring*. Boston: Little, Brown and Company.

Watson, J. (1985a) *Nursing: human science and human care*. Norwalk, Connecticut: Appleton-Century-Crofts.

Watson, J. (1985b) Reflections of different methodologies for the future of nursing. In *Qualitative research methods in nursing*. Edited by M.M. Leininger. Orlando, Florida: Grune & Stratton, 343–349.

Wax, R. (1960) Reciprocity in field work. In *Human organisation research*, Edited by R.N. Adams and J.J. Preiss. Homewood, Illinois: Dorsey, 90–98.

Weatherston, L. (1979) Theory of nursing: creating effective care. *Journal of Advanced Nursing*, 4, 365–375.

White, M. B. (1972) Importance of selected nursing activities. *Nursing Research*, 21:1, 4–13.

Wiedenbach, E. (1964) *Clinical nursing: a helping art*. New York: Springer Publishing Company.

Wilson, H.S. (1985) *Research in nursing*. Menlo Park, California: Addison-Wesley Publishing Company.

Wooldridge, P.J.; Leonard, R.C.; and Skipper, J.K. (1983) Relating behavioural science to nursing science. In *Behavioural science and nursing theory*. Edited by P.J. Wooldridge; M.H. Schmitt; J.K. Skipper; and R.C. Leonard. St.Louis: The C.V.Mosby Company, 5–35.

Wu, R. (1973) *Behaviour and illness*. Englewood Cliffs, New Jersey: Prentice-Hall.

Yura, H. and Walsh, M.B. (1973) *The nursing process*. (2nd ed.). New York: Appleton-Century-Crofts.

Zigarmi, D. and Zigarmi, P. (1979) *The psychological stresses of ethnographic research*. Paper presented at the annual meeting of the American Educational Research Association, Toronto, March 28.

Zimmerman D.S. and Blainey, C.G. (1970) The goal-directed nursing approach: it does work. *American Journal Nursing*, 70:2, 306–310.